MyPlate
for Moms,
How to Feed Yourself & Your Family Better

Elizabeth M. Ward, M.S., R.D.

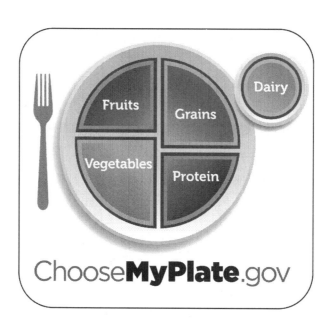

Choose**MyPlate**.gov

Decoding the Dietary Guidelines for Your Real Life

MyPlate for Moms, How to Feed Yourself & Your Family Better
Copyright © 2011 by Elizabeth Ward

ISBN-13: 978-0615528090
ISBN-10: 0615528090

Cover and interior design by Patricia Robinson, patrobinsondesign@mac.com

Cover photo: © Clerkenwell_Images

Nutritional analysis by Elizabeth M. Ward, M.S., R.D.

Other books by Elizabeth M. Ward, M.S., R.D.:

Expect the Best Pregnancy, Your Guide to Healthy Eating Before, During, & After Pregnancy (Wiley 2009)

The Complete Idiot's Guide to Feeding Your Baby and Toddler (Alpha 2008)

Published by Loughlin Press, Reading, MA

For my mom,
who taught me about healthy eating.

CONTENTS

Meet MyPlate

YOU'RE LOOKING FOR A WAY TO EAT BETTER, and the last thing you need in your busy life is time-consuming advice that's difficult to follow and doesn't allow for your favorite foods. MyPlate, the government's newest symbol for good nutrition, provides a simple solution for healthy eating for you and your family. The food pyramid is gone for good, but the message remains the same: Nutritious foods form the basis of good health.

MyPlate is an icon that dishes out visual reminders about what to eat. It's an interpretation of the 2010 Dietary Guidelines for Americans, the federal government's nutritional guidance to promote health and reduce the risk of chronic conditions, such as heart disease and obesity, through better nutrition and regular physical activity.

Healthy eating is typically thought of as an all-or-nothing affair, with no middle ground. But banning the foods you love usually results in feelings of deprivation that cause you to abandon your good intentions. Or, you may just be too busy to think about healthy eating, opting to fly by the seat of your pants instead of planning balanced meals and snacks.

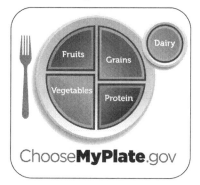

You may feel like you'll never get a grip on your eating habits, or your family's. Take heart. MyPlate can help you and your family to better health right now. Its message is simple: Fill half your plate with fruits and vegetables; about one-quarter of it with grains like pasta, rice, or cereal; and the remainder with protein-rich foods, such as lean meat, poultry, seafood, eggs, legumes, nuts, and seeds. Pour a cup of low-fat (1%) milk or fortified soy beverage, or have an equal amount of yogurt. You're on your way to healthy eating, just like that.

Ease is one of MyPlate's best traits. Flexibility is another. MyPlate is designed to accommodate all kinds of eating patterns for healthy people over the age of two, including pregnant and nursing women. Just as there is no single "American" diet, there is no one recommendation for healthful eating. MyPlate is not a rigid prescription for taking away all the foods you crave. You don't have to give up wine, hot dogs, chips, and cookies, or anything else in the name of good health. While acknowledging that some foods are better than others, MyPlate does not demand dietary perfection.

Ease is one of MyPlate's best traits. Flexibility is another. MyPlate is designed to accommodate all kinds of eating patterns for healthy people over the age of two, including pregnant and nursing women.

What's on MyPlate, and In This Book

MyPlate is supported by several simple messages that you can start working on well before your next meal or snack. There's no need to make all the suggested improvements at once, however. As you read this book, you'll see that it's best to start with one small change and add others as you go along. Here are the top eight ways to start following the MyPlate guidelines:

1. **Enjoy your food, but eat less, and avoid oversized portions.** The size of your plate matters; larger plates often mean larger portions. Most adults should eat less, and some kids may need to reduce serving sizes to help stabilize childhood obesity. Chapters One and Two offer information about calorie balance and weight control for all ages and stages, including adults, pregnant and nursing women, and children. Physical activity plays an important role in weight control and good health. Find out how you can easily get the exercise you need in Chapter Three.

2. **Make half of your plate fruits and vegetables.** Produce provides the nutrients that often go missing in the typical American diet, including potassium and fiber. Plus, fruits and vegetables are filling and nearly all are relatively low in calories. In Chapter Four, you'll discover dozens of easy and creative ways to include an array of produce in your diet, and your family's. In Chapter Nine, you'll find delicious and nutritious recipes for fruit and vegetables.

3. **Make at least half your grains whole grains.** Whole grains have more fiber and other nutrients than highly refined grains, such as white bread, but our whole grain intake is way too low. Chapter Four offers simple strategies for including more whole grains, and Chapter Nine serves up dozens of delicious ways to prepare them.

4. **Switch to fat-free or low-fat (1%) milk.** Fat-free and low-fat (1%) milk have the same amount of protein, vitamins, calcium, and other minerals as higher-fat milks, but with fewer calories and less saturated fat. Milk is a major source of calcium and vitamin D, two nutrients that are often in short supply in our diets. Check out the tips for working in more dairy foods in Chapter Four, and the recipes using milk, yogurt, and cheese in Chapter Nine.

5. **Check the sodium in prepared foods, and choose the foods with lower numbers.** Excess sodium in the diet is linked to high blood pressure. No adult or child should eat more than 2,300 milligrams of sodium a day, and many adults may need far less. Chapter Five provides the low-down on sodium, which includes some high points for this important mineral, and includes ways to flavor foods without salt.

6. **Drink water instead of sugary drinks.** Soda, energy drinks, and sports beverages are major sources of added sugar and calories in our diets, and they offer nothing in the way of nutrition. Discover why added sugar is so problematic in Chapters Five and Eight, and how you can easily slash sugar in your diet.

7. **Eat a variety of protein-rich foods.** For the first time ever, the 2010 Dietary Guidelines recommend eating seafood twice a week in place of meat and poultry, and MyPlate reflects that recommendation. MyPlate also encourages a variety of protein foods, including lean meat, poultry, beans or peas, nuts, soy, and eggs. Learn more about protein in Chapter Seven.

   There's no need to make all the suggested improvements at once... you'll see that it's best to start with one small change and add others as you go along.

8. **Use healthy fats.** Fats aren't an official MyPlate food group, but they are part of your diet. Learn which fats are better for you in Chapter Six, and what you should consider about cholesterol.

Healthy Eating Begins at Home

As a registered dietitian and working mother of three, I know how hard it is to keep yourself, and your family, on track for healthy eating and regular physical activity. Time is tight. And, it's not always possible to block out what the 2010 Dietary Guidelines for Americans calls our "obesogenic environment," that promotes poor foods choices and inadequate physical activity.

At times, it can feel like you're fighting a losing battle against the smell of French fries wafting from that popular fast food joint as you drive by, chocolate chip cookies that are bigger than your hand, and the candy bar calling your name at the check-out counter. It's tough for adults to resist the temptation of readily-available food that smells and tastes delicious, and it's even harder for kids.

With the help of MyPlate, you decide what to eat and drink, and how much to exercise. It may seem like the odds are stacked against you when it comes to healthier habits, but never give up trying to improve on what happens in your own home. You can't control the number of burger joints or pizza places in your town, but you can control whether you offer tater tots or the better alternative, a baked potato, to your child; the portion size of high calorie foods you put on MyPlate; and how much physical activity you and your family get.

You've got a lot on your plate already. That's why this book is set up to deliver tips you can use in a flash, and allows you to read more about good nutrition and exercise when you have the time.

I AM INDEBTED to my editor and to my designer for helping me bring my first self-published book to fruition. They went the extra mile to help, offering valuable advice and meeting impossible deadlines. I am lucky to know them, and I am grateful for their experience, patience, and expertise. Thanks, too, to Hillary Wright, M.Ed., R.D., and Alanna Levine, M.D., for reviewing *MyPlate for Moms*. As always, I need to thank my family for putting up with me while I wrote this book. I promise to make it up to you!

CHAPTER 1

MyPlate for a Healthy Weight

MOTHERS and other busy people often wish for a balanced life with fewer chores, less work, and more time spent relaxing with family and friends. Achieving balance in any area of life is no mean feat. It takes vigilance to monitor yourself so that you don't take on too many projects, forgo regular exercise, raid the kitchen every night, or all of the above!

It's not always easy to achieve, but balance is a worthy goal. Balance is the cornerstone of your good health, and your family's.

When it comes to healthy eating, calorie balance is one of the major messages in the 2010 Dietary Guidelines for Americans. With its practical, easy-to-understand suggestions about what, and how much, to eat, MyPlate echoes the guidelines' recommendations to avoid oversized servings.

Calorie balance is all about equalizing the energy from the foods and beverages you eat with the calories you burn through everyday living and physical activity. The goal of calorie balance is achieving and maintaining a healthy weight, which helps you to be more energetic and to avoid chronic conditions, including heart disease and diabetes.

With all the talk of tallying fat grams, cutting carbohydrates, and boosting protein intake as ways to lose weight, the importance of calories in the weight-control equation is often cast aside. Yet, calorie balance is the linchpin of losing pounds or maintaining your weight within a healthy range.

Calorie Balance: Take It Personally

The calorie balance concept is simple: To maintain weight, eat as many calories as you burn. You'll put on pounds if your calorie consumption consistently exceeds your needs, and you'll lose weight when you eat fewer calories than you expend.

Calorie balance is not a one-size-fits-all concept. It's personal, and it changes with age, and with different stages of life.

Calculating your calorie "budget" is the first step to a better diet no matter what your weight goal. Once your calorie quota is clear, you're on your way to knowing how much energy you have to "spend" on the nutrient-rich foods MyPlate recommends.

You may be thinking, "Now I have a calorie budget I have to stick to?" That's fair. It may seem like there's yet another task on your to-do list. Once you discover why calorie balance matters, and how you can better achieve it for yourself and your family, it becomes second nature when choosing what to eat at meals and snacks.

An Ounce of Prevention Is Worth a Pound of Cure

As anyone who has ever tried to shed extra pounds knows, it's far easier to prevent becoming overweight than it is to remedy the situation. Reducing your body weight to a healthy range requires significant effort—one that you probably would rather avoid. That's why the Dietary Guidelines strongly recommend preventing excess pounds in adults, and fostering healthy weight gain in children, which is no simple task.

Seventy-two percent of American men and 64% of American women are overweight, and one-third of all U.S. adults are obese. The growing incidence of excess weight and obesity among American children is a pressing problem that the Dietary Guidelines address with a sense of urgency. That's because about 32% of children and teens ages two to 19 years old are overweight and 17% of them are considered obese. (See page 19 for more on healthy eating for kids.)

No one is certain of the long-term health effects of childhood obesity, but we do know that excess pounds increase the risk of chronic conditions in adults, including the following:

- Heart disease
- High blood pressure
- Type 2 diabetes
- Certain types of cancer

In addition to a greater chance for debilitating chronic conditions, carrying around extra fat weighs you down in other ways that affect quality of life. Along with a poor diet, excess weight saps your energy, may disturb your sleep, and could keep you from pursuing hobbies and other activities, such as regular exercise.

Are you overweight?

You complain about your "muffin top." Maybe your "thunder thighs" or "bra bulge" annoy you. If you think you need to lose weight, you may be right. But it's not enough to jump on the scale and decide that slimming down is in order.

Height is associated with weight, but no single weight is the healthiest for your height. Rather, there is a healthy range for each height. Body Mass Index (BMI) is the most accurate way to determine whether your weight falls within the healthy range. BMI assesses body fat based on height and weight. (If you're pregnant, use your pre-pregnancy weight to figure BMI.)

Generally speaking, BMI is a reliable indicator of extra fat. However, no method is perfect, and BMI has at least one known fault: it makes very muscular people seem like they have too much fat. Given the statistics on Americans who are overweight and obese in the United States, BMI's major pitfall won't affect most people.

To determine BMI, you'll need to know your exact height and weight. Jump on the scale first thing in the morning, after using the bathroom, and before eating or drinking anything. Once you have the necessary information, check the chart on page 4 to find out if your weight is within the healthy range.

How did you do? If your weight is considered healthy, your calorie consumption is on track for now. But you're not necessarily off the hook. Your calories are in balance, but your diet may not be. A healthy body weight does not guarantee that you're including enough calcium, vitamin D, potassium, fiber, and other nutrients found lacking in the American diet by the Dietary Guidelines. (See page 49 for more on how to get the nutrients you need.)

If your BMI is in the overweight or obese range, you're eating too many calories. To lose weight, you need to cut back on calories, become more physically active, or better yet, a combination of the two.

Body Mass Index Table

BMI	Normal						Overweight					Obese										Extreme Obesity															
Height (inches)	19	20	21	22	23	24	25	26	27	28	29	30	31	32	33	34	35	36	37	38	39	40	41	42	43	44	45	46	47	48	49	50	51	52	53	54
												Body Weight (pounds)																								
58	91	96	100	105	110	115	119	124	129	134	138	143	148	153	158	162	167	172	177	181	186	191	196	201	205	210	215	220	224	229	234	239	244	248	253	258
59	94	99	104	109	114	119	124	128	133	138	143	148	153	158	163	168	173	178	183	188	193	198	203	208	212	217	222	227	232	237	242	247	252	257	262	267
60	97	102	107	112	118	123	128	133	138	143	148	153	158	163	168	174	179	184	189	194	199	204	209	215	220	225	230	235	240	245	250	255	261	266	271	276
61	100	106	111	116	122	127	132	137	143	148	153	158	164	169	174	180	185	190	195	201	206	211	217	222	227	232	238	243	248	254	259	264	269	275	280	285
62	104	109	115	120	126	131	136	142	147	153	158	164	169	175	180	186	191	196	202	207	213	218	224	229	235	240	246	251	256	262	267	273	278	284	289	295
63	107	113	118	124	130	135	141	146	152	158	163	169	175	180	186	191	197	203	208	214	220	225	231	237	242	248	254	259	265	270	278	282	287	293	299	304
64	110	116	122	128	134	140	145	151	157	163	169	174	180	186	192	197	204	209	215	221	227	232	238	244	250	256	262	267	273	279	285	291	296	302	308	314
65	114	120	126	132	138	144	150	156	162	168	174	180	186	192	198	204	210	216	222	228	234	240	246	252	258	264	270	276	282	288	294	300	306	312	318	324
66	118	124	130	136	142	148	155	161	167	173	179	186	192	198	204	210	216	223	229	235	241	247	253	260	266	272	278	284	291	297	303	309	315	322	328	334
67	121	127	134	140	146	153	159	166	172	178	185	191	198	204	211	217	223	230	236	242	249	255	261	268	274	280	287	293	299	306	312	319	325	331	338	344
68	125	131	138	144	151	158	164	171	177	184	190	197	203	210	216	223	230	236	243	249	256	262	269	276	282	289	295	302	308	315	322	328	335	341	348	354
69	128	135	142	149	155	162	169	176	182	189	196	203	209	216	223	230	236	243	250	257	263	270	277	284	291	297	304	311	318	324	331	338	345	351	358	365
70	132	139	146	153	160	167	174	181	188	195	202	209	216	222	229	236	243	250	257	264	271	278	285	292	299	306	313	320	327	334	341	348	355	362	369	376
71	136	143	150	157	165	172	179	186	193	200	208	215	222	229	236	243	250	257	265	272	279	286	293	301	308	315	322	329	338	343	351	358	365	372	379	386
72	140	147	154	162	169	177	184	191	199	206	213	221	228	235	242	250	258	265	272	279	287	294	302	309	316	324	331	338	346	353	361	368	375	383	390	397
73	144	151	159	166	174	182	189	197	204	212	219	227	235	242	250	257	265	272	280	288	295	302	310	318	325	333	340	348	355	363	371	378	386	393	401	408
74	148	155	163	171	179	186	194	202	210	218	225	233	241	249	256	264	272	280	287	295	303	311	319	326	334	342	350	358	365	373	381	389	396	404	412	420
75	152	160	168	176	184	192	200	208	216	224	232	240	248	256	264	272	279	287	295	303	311	319	327	335	343	351	359	367	375	383	391	399	407	415	423	431
76	156	164	172	180	189	197	205	213	221	230	238	246	254	263	271	279	287	295	304	312	320	328	336	344	353	361	369	377	385	394	402	410	418	426	435	443

Source: Adapted from Clinical Guidelines on the Identification, Evaluation, and Treatment of Overweight and Obesity in Adults: The Evidence Report.

○ MYPLATE FOR MOMS, HOW TO FEED YOURSELF & YOUR FAMILY BETTER

BMI is for use in people ages two and older, but between two and 18 years, a child's BMI must be considered along with his age. (See page 20 for more on figuring out a child's BMI.)

Calculating Calories

Measuring your BMI provides a goal: weight gain, maintenance, or weight loss. Now, you need to personalize an eating plan to help you reach your goal. It's easier to craft an eating plan that includes the foods you need for good health when you know how many calories you have to work with. Calorie needs are affected by three main factors:

1. Physical Activity:
The Dietary Guidelines divide physical activity into three levels to help determine calorie needs. Pick the one that best describes you:
- *Sedentary:* You perform the bare minimum of physical activity to get through a typical day.
- *Moderately active:* You include physical activity that is equivalent to walking 1.5 to 3 miles every day at the rate of 3 to 4 miles an hour, (about 15 minutes to 20 minutes per mile) in addition to the light activity you perform in a typical day.
- *Active:* You walk more than 3 miles a day at a rate of 15 minutes per mile to 20 minutes per mile (3 to 4 miles an hour) or the equivalent, in addition to the light physical activity you would do to get through a typical day.

The more you move around, the more you're able to eat to maintain, or lose weight. It's important to be honest with yourself about your physical activity level because it plays a big role in calorie needs. Be careful not to overestimate calorie expenditure, or you may be confused and disappointed that weight loss or weight control doesn't come easier to you. (See page 33 for more on the benefits of physical activity and easy ways to become more active for you and your family.)

2. Age:
As you get older, your resting metabolism—the number of calories your body burns to maintain basic functions, such as breathing and digestion, slows down. The changes are gradual and they typically start in your mid-20s.

Lean tissue, which is mostly muscle, starts to wane in men and women, and the rise in total body fat begins. As you lose lean tissue, which requires more calories to sustain than fat, daily calorie needs decline, too.

Continue to eat the same number of calories without increasing the calories you expend through physical activity or by increasing muscle mass, and you will gain weight. Exercise that builds or maintains muscle mass, such as resistance training, promotes a faster metabolic rate.

3. Gender:

Generally speaking, men burn more calories on a pound for pound basis because they have more muscle. A woman's metabolic "engine" is slower because she has more fat tissue.

How many calories for you?

You know your age and gender, and you've picked a physical activity category: you're either sedentary, moderately active, or active. You're ready to find out how many calories you need each day.

The following chart estimates daily calorie needs to maintain your current weight, estimated being the operative word.

The chart provided in the 2010 Dietary Guidelines, uses average heights and healthy weight for adults. The government's reference adult man measures 5'10" tall and weighs 154 pounds, while the reference woman is 5'4" and tips the scales at 126 pounds. Does that describe you or anyone you know to the letter? Probably not, but that's OK. (You can also find out your daily calorie needs to maintain, gain, or lose weight at ChooseMyPlate.gov. Click on Interactive Tools and enter the information requested.)

While very few of us fit the exact description of the reference man or woman, you can imagine why it's necessary to have them: It's enormously difficult to determine the daily calorie needs for millions of adults. When it comes to kids, there is even more estimating going on, because of the wide variation in reference heights

Estimated Calorie Needs per Day by Age, Gender, and Physical Activity Level

Estimated amounts of calories[a] needed to maintain calorie balance for various gender and age groups at three different levels of physical activity. The estimates are rounded to the nearest 200 calories. An individual's calorie needs may be higher or lower than these average estimates.

Gender/ Activity level [b]	Male/ Sedentary	Male/ Moderately Active	Male/ Active	Female[c]/ Sedentary	Female[c]/ Moderately Active	Female[c]/ Active
Age (years)						
2	1,000	1,000	1,000	1,000	1,000	1,000
3	1,200	1,400	1,400	1,000	1,200	1,400
4	1,200	1,400	1,600	1,200	1,400	1,400
5	1,200	1,400	1,600	1,200	1,400	1,600
6	1,400	1,600	1,800	1,200	1,400	1,600
7	1,400	1,600	1,800	1,200	1,600	1,800
8	1,400	1,600	2,000	1,400	1,600	1,800
9	1,600	1,800	2,000	1,400	1,600	1,800
10	1,600	1,800	2,200	1,400	1,800	2,000
11	1,800	2,000	2,200	1,600	1,800	2,000
12	1,800	2,200	2,400	1,600	2,000	2,200
13	2,000	2,200	2,600	1,600	2,000	2,200
14	2,000	2,400	2,800	1,800	2,000	2,400
15	2,200	2,600	3,000	1,800	2,000	2,400
16	2,400	2,800	3,200	1,800	2,000	2,400
17	2,400	2,800	3,200	1,800	2,000	2,400
18	2,400	2,800	3,200	1,800	2,000	2,400
19–20	2,600	2,800	3,000	2,000	2,200	2,400
21–25	2,400	2,800	3,000	2,000	2,200	2,400
26–30	2,400	2,600	3,000	1,800	2,000	2,400
31–35	2,400	2,600	3,000	1,800	2,000	2,200
36–40	2,400	2,600	2,800	1,800	2,000	2,200
41–45	2,200	2,600	2,800	1,800	2,000	2,200
46–50	2,200	2,400	2,800	1,800	2,000	2,200
51–55	2,200	2,400	2,800	1,600	1,800	2,200
56–60	2,200	2,400	2,600	1,600	1,800	2,200
61–65	2,000	2,400	2,600	1,600	1,800	2,000
66–70	2,000	2,200	2,600	1,600	1,800	2,000
71–75	2,000	2,200	2,600	1,600	1,800	2,000
76+	2,000	2,200	2,200	1,600	1,800	2,000

a. Based on Estimated Energy Requirements (EER) equations, using reference heights (average) and reference weights (healthy) for each age-gender group. For children and adolescents, reference height and weight vary. For adults, the reference man is 5 feet 10 inches tall and weighs 154 pounds. The reference woman is 5 feet 4 inches tall and weighs 126 pounds. EER equations are from the Institute of Medicine. Dietary Reference Intakes for Energy, Carbohydrate, Fiber, Fat, Fatty Acids, Cholesterol, Protein, and Amino Acids. Washington (DC): The National Academies Press; 2002.
b. Sedentary means a lifestyle that includes only the light physical activity associated with typical day-to-day life. Moderately active means a lifestyle that includes physical activity equivalent to walking about 1.5 to 3 miles per day at 3 to 4 miles per hour, in addition to the light physical activity associated with typical day-to-day life. Active means a lifestyle that includes physical activity equivalent to walking more than 3 miles per day at 3 to 4 miles per hour, in addition to the light physical activity associated with typical day-to-day life.
c. Estimates for females do not include women who are pregnant or breastfeeding.

Source: Britten P, Marcoe K, Yamini S, Davis C. Development of food intake patterns for the MyPyramid Food Guidance System. J Nutr Educ Behav 2006;38(6 Suppl):S78-S92.

and weights. In spite of its shortcomings, the Dietary Guideline's calorie chart serves as a solid starting point for figuring calorie needs for people ages two to 102. If you don't choose the calorie level given to you at ChooseMyPlate.gov for weight loss or weight gain, you can make your own adjustments based on the chart. Pregnant and nursing women can find out how many calories they need by clicking on Pregnant & Breastfeeding at ChooseMyPlate.gov.

The Weight Loss Equation

Now you're clear on the number of calories you need to achieve your personal weight goal. Keep that number in mind when you choose what to eat, and weight control becomes a lot easier.

You don't have to slash calories to the bare minimum or exercise for hours every day to get results. Few people have the resources, time, or motivation to drastically alter their lifestyles, even if it means feeling better now and reducing their risk for chronic conditions in the long run. It's better to personalize a lifestyle program that works for you and your family.

Just about anybody can lose weight when they put their mind to it; people do it every day. What most people fail to master is maintaining a healthy weight, and doing so by eating a balanced diet that provides the nutrients they need along with regular physical activity.

A very low calorie diet will slim you down fast. But scaling back too much allows hunger to get the upper hand, causing motivated waist-watchers to call it quits and revert to unhealthy eating habits. Most people want a quick fix to a weight problem that's been in the making for years, and possibly, decades. A slower, more measured approach to curbing calories allows you to adopt healthier habits that have a greater chance of sticking with you. For example, cutting 100 calories a day—the amount found in a medium chocolate chip cookie, one tablespoon of butter, or about an ounce of potato chips—without changing your activity level can trim five pounds from your frame in just six months. The best part? You won't feel deprived.

It's even better to combine calorie reduction with increased physical activity to improve your chances of lasting weight loss and better health. For example, reducing your calorie intake by 100 a day, as described above, and burning an additional 150 calories daily through physical activity will help you to lose upwards of two pounds a month, or about 12 pounds in six-month's time. That may not sound like much progress, but since the changes to your life would be nearly imperceptible, they'd be easier to maintain in the long run, which is what counts the most.

If you're after a faster rate of weight loss, you could lower your daily calorie consumption by 500. Or, you could eat 250 fewer calories and work off another 250 with additional physical activity. Whatever strategy you use, don't eat fewer than 1,600 calories a day. It's difficult to get the nutrients you need on a very low calorie diet, and you may feel so hungry that you abandon your efforts to eat better and exercise on a regular basis.

What if you suspect your child is overweight? See page 20 for more on calorie balance for kids.

Where Calories Come From

You have a calorie budget to help you lose weight, maintain it, or gain it. That number is useless if you're clueless about where calories come from. Understanding the energy sources in foods is helpful when reading food labels, and is a must for improving calorie balance.

There are four sources of calories: carbohydrate, protein, fat, and alcohol.

Carbohydrates supply four calories per gram. They are the primary source of energy for most Americans. Carbohydrates can be *simple*, a category that includes sugar, or *complex*, including starches and dietary fiber.

Sugars are found naturally in foods, including milk and yogurt. Sugars, such as sucrose (table sugar) and high-fructose corn syrup, are often added to foods, such as

> ☐ **Calorie Balance for Pregnant and Nursing Women**
>
> Pregnant women who begin their pregnancy at a Body Mass Index (BMI) within the normal range need about 330 more calories every day starting in the second trimester than they do when they are not expecting. Women who are in the underweight, overweight, or obese ranges should consult with their health-care provider and a registered dietitian (R.D.) about the number of extra calories that is right for them. You need about the same number of calories when breastfeeding as you do in the third trimester of pregnancy. Pregnant and nursing women should choose nutrient-rich foods, such as whole grains, lean sources of protein, fruits, vegetables, beans, and nuts to get the calories and other nutrients they need to nourish their children, and themselves.

carbonated soft drinks. Fiber is found naturally in foods, and may be used as an ingredient in packaged foods, too.

When it comes to carbs, there's really only one rule. Choose foods with naturally-occurring carbohydrates, such as whole-grain breads and breakfast cereals, vegetables, and beans more often, and limit refined grains, including white bread and crackers, as well as foods with added sugars, like sweet beverages, cookies, and ice cream.

Protein also provides four calories per gram. The body breaks down the protein in foods into amino acids, the raw materials used to build and preserve muscle and tissues, and to make every substance in the body. A wide variety of animal and plant foods provide protein, including meat, dairy, eggs, seafood, beans, nuts, seeds, and soy products.

MyPlate recommends mixing it up when it comes to protein foods. Select lean protein-packed foods to get the protein you need with a minimum of extra calories.

Fats supply nine calories per gram. You need fat for the energy and essential fatty acids (EFA) it provides. Your body cannot produce EFA, compounds central to good health, so it must get them from food.

Four types of fat are found naturally in food, and in packaged foods: saturated, trans, monounsaturated, and polyunsaturated. All fats contain the same number of calories but have different effects on your health. Make the majority of fat you eat the unsaturated type, which comes primarily from seafood, nuts, seeds, and oils.

Alcohol offers seven calories per gram (not counting the mixers). Alcohol is one of the top calorie

⬛ Be a Calorie Sleuth

The Nutrition Facts label is a boon to calorie counters. In 1994, all manufacturers were required to include a Nutrition Facts Panel on their products. The label applies to all packaged foods regulated by the Food and Drug Administration (FDA). It does not apply to all food products, however. Meat, poultry, and seafood products are exempt because the United States Department of Agriculture (USDA) regulates them.

The Nutrition Facts panel provides information about the calories and other nutrients in one portion of food. You need to be careful when reading the Nutrition Facts label. It's not designed to be tricky, but there may be more than one portion in a food container. For example, some juice drinks provide two or more servings in what appears to be a single-serve container. If you drink more than one portion, you need to account for the calories.

contributors in adult Americans' diets. The calorie content of alcoholic beverages vary based on the alcohol content, and whether the alcohol is mixed with juice or other soft drinks, milk, or cream.

Simple Swaps that Save Calories

One of MyPlate's messages is to enjoy your food, but don't eat too much.

Here are some easy ways to cut calories throughout your day, without really altering your eating routine. Many of these small changes will also naturally decrease the amount of solid fats, added sugar, sodium, and refined grains you eat while increasing your intake of calcium, vitamin D, potassium, and fiber, four of the nutrients the 2010 Dietary Guidelines say we need more of.

Instead of:	Eat this:	Save this many calories:
2 slices stuffed crust pizza	2 slices thin crust pizza	404
Milk chocolate candy bar (1.3 oz.)	100-calorie frozen fudge bar	102
Large chocolate chip cookie (2 oz.)	1 small chocolate chip cookie (1 oz.)	133
Single-serve bag of snack chips (1.5 oz.)	3 cups microwave popcorn, 50% less fat	75
Plain bagel (4 oz.) with 2 tablespoons regular cream cheese	Whole-wheat bagel (1 oz.) with 1 tablespoon peanut butter	284
Large caffe latte (20 oz.) made with full-fat milk	Large caffe latte (20 oz.) made with fat-free milk	120
Ice cream frappe (16 oz.)	Smoothie made with banana and fat-free milk	450

Source: Manufacturer data; USDA; MyFood-a-pedia, www.myfoodapedia.gov.

The Calorie Balance Conundrum

You're on the path to better, more balanced eating, then it happens. Life trips you up by placing temptation square in your path, and you give into it. No worries! Dietary disasters happen to everybody, including nutrition experts.

The key to lasting weight control is figuring out what triggers your overeating and how to get the upper hand so that you are in control of your appetite. Here are some of the most common reasons for calorie overload and how to prevent them from getting the best of your motivation to eat better.

☐ **Problem #1: Portion Distortion.** If a half box of pasta is your idea of a serving, or you think a typical bagel is the caloric equivalent of one piece of bread, you're way off base. You've got lots of company!

It's safe to say that most of us are out of touch with what health experts hold up as healthy portions. Otherwise, we wouldn't be struggling with our weight. MyPlate recommends avoiding oversized portions, but you may not know what reasonable portions are, particularly if you've been serving yourself and your family large portions for a long time. It's important to pay attention to suggested serving sizes because even slightly more than you should have of healthy foods, including bread, cereals, and oils, can add up to hundreds of extra calories a day, thwarting your best attempts at weight control.

☑ **Solution:** Many fruits, including an apple, small banana, a pear, an orange, and kiwi, come in perfectly portioned packages. So do eggs. Other foods need to be weighed and measured or at least "eyeballed" so that you get the portions right. Use smaller plates and bowls, and taller glasses to cut back on food. Downsizing dinnerware means serving yourself less without feeling cheated. Taller glasses trick you into thinking you're drinking more. MyPlate offers up the right serving size in each food group. If you want to know the full details about proper serving sizes from each food group, go to Choose MyPlate.gov for helpful lists.

☐ **Problem #2: You skimp on meals, or skip them.** News Flash: You need to eat to lose weight. Regular meals and snacks that fit into your calorie budget are the backbone of easier weight control. Skipping or skimping on food slows down your metabolism, causing you to burn fewer calories. It also sets you up to lose control at your next meal as extreme hunger may prompt you to eat more calories than you need.

☑ **Solution:** Make time to eat, or bring food with you to eat in the car or at the office. Meal quality matters, of course. The best meals and snacks include protein and fiber to help you feel fuller for longer. When you skimp on breakfast, you lose out on several nutrients, including calcium, vitamin D, potassium, and fiber.

Generally speaking, people who've lost weight and kept it off eat breakfast every day. Breakfast is especially important because it provides an edge in keeping pounds at bay, as it appears to curb calorie consumption for the remainder of the day. Include protein and fiber at breakfast. One study found that people who ate a meal with two eggs at least five times a week took in, on average, 300 fewer calories during the rest of the day, compared to those who noshed on a bagel meal of the same caloric value. Other healthy breakfast ideas: whole-grain cereal, low-fat (1%) milk, and fruit; or two slices whole-grain toast topped with low-fat cream cheese and 2 ounces smoked salmon with a cup of berries. On the go? Grab a carton of fat-free Greek yogurt, small whole-grain roll, and fruit. At work, microwave quick-cooking oatmeal with fat-free or low-fat (1%) milk and top with ¼ cup California raisins.

☐ **Problem #3: You're sleep deprived.** Like so many busy people, you don't get enough ZZZ's. Lack of sleep could be affecting your weight, and your child's, in more ways than one. Experts say sleep deprivation plays havoc with your metabolism because it disturbs the hormones that keep hunger and satiety (eating satisfaction) in check. When you feel sleepy during the day, it's likely that you'll reach for food, or drinks, that provide a quick shot of energy, including those that are high in sugar, caffeine, or both, which may help you temporarily fight off fatigue. However, your calorie balance may remain out of whack in the long run. And, if you're relying on caffeine to get you through the day, it's difficult to break the cycle you're in because you may not be able to get the rest you need.

☑ **Solution:** Hit the sack earlier, and insure a better quality of sleep by avoiding caffeine in the afternoon and large meals or snacks and alcohol at night. Sleeping for the recommended seven to eight hours a night is no magic bullet for weight control, but it helps by normalizing your metabolism and by energizing you enough to care about shopping for healthy ingredients, making nutritious meals, and working out on a regular basis.

☐ **Problem #4: Special events.** Valentine's Day, birthday celebrations, and barbecues—there's always some event to test your dietary resolve. It's OK to save up a few hundred calories here and there to splurge on a special occasion or major holiday, but keep close tabs on your eating. You may think you have more calories in reserve than you do, causing you to overdo it.

☑ **Solution:** Before any party or celebration, fortify yourself with a snack, such as low-fat yogurt or cottage cheese combined with fruit or whole-grain crackers, to blunt your hunger. At the gathering, splurge sensibly. Decide on one or two foods to try, and take tiny portions. The first few bites are the most satisfying so there's no point in eating more. Stop eating when you are satisfied, not full.

☐ **Problem #5: Weekends.** Weekends come around every six days, and they often spell trouble for weight control. Regarding Saturday and Sunday (and sometimes Friday!) as days off from healthy eating can easily erase the achievements you make during the week. Researchers who tracked food intake of 48 people ages 50 to 60 years old found they consumed an average of 236 more calories on Saturdays than during the week—the equivalent of nine pounds of body fat in a year's time.

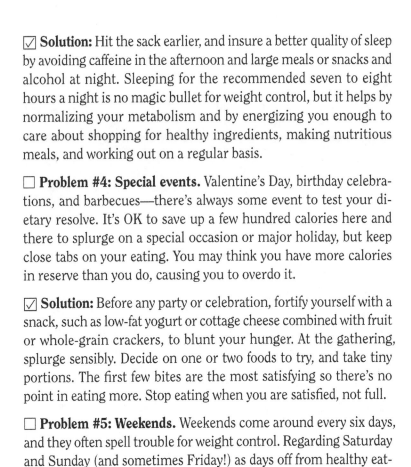

☐ **Chew Gum, Eat Less?**

Pop a piece of gum before reaching for a snack, and you'll likely consume fewer calories. Gum chewing is a great way to occupy your mouth and the chewing may help to relieve the frazzled nerves you typically soothe with food.

☑ **Solution:** Sidestep weekend temptations by jumping on the scale every Friday morning and again on Monday. Use the extra time on weekends to sleep (which benefits your metabolism) and to be more physically active with your family and friends. When you indulge, don't waste calories on foods or drinks you don't absolutely love, and try to keep portions on the smaller side.

☐ **Problem #6: Mindless munching**. Can't remember what you ate five minutes ago? You may suffer from "eating amnesia," an unofficial condition that makes you forget inhaling lunch in your mini-van, eating your child's leftovers, and polishing off a pint of ice cream while watching TV.

☑ **Solution:** Eat on a regular basis and include protein and fiber at every meal and snack to keep you fuller for longer. That way, you won't be tempted to nibble, or worse. Keep a food log and write down everything that passes your lips to highlight potential dietary disasters. When you eat, sit down at a table and focus on what you're doing. The 2010 Dietary Guidelines calls out TV watching as a reason for overeating and cautions us to avoid combining the two activities. If you insist on eating while watching television, portion out a small serving, and do not bring the entire package of chips or cookies or the container of ice cream into the TV room.

☐ **Problem #7: You deny yourself treats.** Deprivation is the Achilles heel of any well-intentioned eating plan, so avoid all-out sacrifice. While there are no forbidden foods, you must account for what you eat.

☑ **Solution:** Adults can include about 100-calorie's worth of treats as part of your overall daily calorie allowance; children can have more in accordance with their calorie needs. It's easier to keep calories in check with 100-calorie frozen treats such as fudge bars or ice cream cups, and portion-controlled bags of chips or cookies. Save money by dividing up bigger packages of healthy snack foods, such as pretzels, into 100-calorie portions.

☐ **Problem #8: Dining Out.** You're trying to eat less, but you like to dine out. Maybe you have to eat away from home often for reasons other than relaxation and fun. Restaurant fare can take a toll on your waistline because it almost always dishes up more calories, fat, and sodium and less fiber than what you make at home, and the bigger portions restaurants serve tempt you to eat more.

☑ **Solution:** Investigate the calories of the dishes you order most often by asking the establishment for nutrition information or go

MyPlate Dines Out

- **Identify restaurants with lighter, healthier fare,** including grilled lean meat, poultry, and seafood.
- **When you're with a crowd, order first.** It sets the tone for the meal, and reduces your temptation to have what they're having.
- **Choose smaller portions or lower-calorie dishes.** For example, order two lower-calorie appetizers, such as shrimp cocktail and broth-based soup instead of a fattier entrée.
- **Order fat-free or low-fat (1%) milk or water instead of a regular soda.**
- **Split an entrée or bring home half of your dinner.** Ask for a doggy bag at the beginning of the meal to prevent you from picking at food that you don't need.
- **Take one piece of bread,** and ask the waiter to take the bread basket off the table. This helps you resist temptation to have another roll, or two.
- **Begin your meal with a garden salad with very little salad dressing or a bowl of broth-based soup.** This helps to curb your appetite.
- **Order an extra side of vegetables that have been steamed or roasted.**
- **Opt for steamed, grilled, or broiled dishes** instead foods smothered in sauces, butter, or oil.
- **Wait until your meal arrives to order alcohol.** You'll down fewer calories overall. Plus, eating is more pleasurable when you're alert and oriented. Leave less room for booze by sipping water, club soda, or a diet soft drink before and during meals.
- **Skip all-you-can-eat buffets,** as they encourage overeating.
- **Order fruit for dessert.**
- **Split high-calorie desserts with as many people as possible.** It may only take one or two bites to satisfy you.

online to get the information. Healthier choices can save you hundreds of calories each time you dine. Play close attention to portions. When you're served too much food, take home half for lunch or dinner the next day. Doggy bags save calories, and money, too. Bringing your own breakfast, lunch, and snacks for when you're away from home cuts down on dining out and is easier on your calorie budget and your pocketbook.

○ MYPLATE FOR MOMS, HOW TO FEED YOURSELF & YOUR FAMILY BETTER

◯ Visualize Proper Portion Sizes

Weighing and measuring foods and drinks is central to controlling portion sizes. You can't bring your food scale and measuring cups and spoons everywhere, so when you're without the tools you use at home, these visual cues will help you determine the right portions.

This amount of food	Looks like this
3 ounces cooked meat, poultry, or fish	A deck of playing cards
1 cup fruit or vegetables	Two small fists
½ cup cooked pasta, rice, or breakfast cereal	A small fist
1 ounce cheese, 1 tablespoon butter, oil, salad dressing, or margarine	Your thumb
1 teaspoon margarine, butter, salad dressing, or oil	The space from the tip of your thumb to the first knuckle

That's a Wrap

Calories and physical activity are critical to good health, but an increasing amount of research suggests that the quality of your diet matters when it comes to weight control, too. That's why most of the remainder of this book is devoted to helping you, and your family, to eat better by including nutrient-rich foods in your everyday life. Next up is calorie balance for kids.

CHAPTER 2

MyPlate for Kids and Moms to Be

HIGH BLOOD PRESSURE, elevated blood cholesterol, and type 2 diabetes are for adults right? Not so much anymore. Chronic conditions once reserved for adulthood are rapidly become more prevalent among teens and younger children. Excess body fat and a poor diet are to blame.

From the early 1970s to 2008, obesity among kids ages 12 to 19 years tripled, and it increased five-fold in six to 11 year-olds. More younger children than ever are overweight, too: where five percent of our toddlers and preschoolers were once considered obese, now 10% of them have body fat levels that are alarmingly high.

For the first time in the history of the Dietary Guidelines, the 2010 version strongly emphasizes the importance of a healthy body weight and balanced diet for kids, and with good reason. Children and teens who are overweight tend to become overweight adults who have great difficulty reaching a healthy weight and maintaining it. In addition, inadequate diets put children at risk for common chronic conditions, whether or not they're overweight.

Children and teens who are overweight tend to become overweight adults who have great difficulty reaching a healthy weight and maintaining it.

The harmful effects of being overweight are harder on the body when developed earlier in life. Right now, childhood obesity is such a serious health threat that the current generation of American children may be the first who *fail* to outlive their parents.

As the Dietary Guidelines aptly point out, preventing becoming overweight and obese is easier than trying to "cure" it years later. Ending the childhood obesity crisis, or at least putting a dent in it, requires the collective efforts of government, industry, schools, and communities. Ultimately, individuals make their own choices about what to eat and to serve the children in their care. That means there's plenty that parents and other caregivers can do to improve a child's diet and lifestyle. Read on for how to help children achieve calorie balance while getting the nutrients they need to thrive, and go on to become healthy adults.

Overweight Children: The Blame Game

When it comes to our childhood obesity predicament, thoughts turn to whom or what to blame for the problem. It's tempting to single out certain foods or ingredients for ballooning waistlines in kids, and in adults. The high fructose corn syrup used to sweeten soft drinks, candy, and other treats is often seen as a major culprit. And while foods sweetened with high fructose corn syrup, and other foods, often contribute excess calories, it's unreasonable to think that one or two foods or ingredients are why American kids are so heavy. Rather, it's a combination of factors that boils down to a singular problem: A calorie balance equation that's out of whack.

Overweight kids consume more calories than they need for normal growth. Their sedentary habits figure prominently into accumulating excess pounds, too. To make matters worse, American children, including kids at a healthy weight, are coming up short for several nutrients that may hamper their development and further boost their risk for chronic conditions.

Is your child overweight?

Your toddler may be plump, and you're wondering if he has a weight problem. Your pediatrician can tell you for sure.

At age two, doctors start measuring your child's Body Mass Index (BMI) and plotting it on a chart that also accounts for your child's age. Unlike people 18 years and older, a child's age must be considered before making a determination about his level of fatness. You can figure your child's BMI at http://apps.nccd.cdc.gov/dnpabmi/ and ask your pediatrician or nurse how best to interpret the results.

If you think your child is overweight, do not put her on a diet. Children are not miniature adults. A child's needs for certain nutrients, including protein, are higher on a pound-for-pound basis than an adult's, and kids need to gain weight to grow and develop properly. It's unwise to drastically restrict a child's calories, but it's OK to offer fat-free and low-fat (1%) milk instead of soft drinks and to limit candy, cookies, and chips. Children ages 12 months to two years need full-fat milk for the calories, fat, and cholesterol it provides, but after age two, most children can drink low-fat (1%) milk or fat-free milk. Overweight children and teens must maintain calorie balance with a healthy diet to support normal growth and development without promoting excess weight gain. Get specific feeding advice from your pediatrician or a registered dietitian (R.D.).

 ## What to do when it's more than "baby fat"?

Helping kids eat a balanced diet that promotes a healthy weight is not easy, especially when they clamor for foods that are relatively high in calories (and low in nutrients), including chicken nuggets, hot dogs, and macaroni and cheese. Children also tend to avoid fruits and vegetables at all costs, and turn up their noses at low-fat milk and yogurt.

Here's what to do if your pediatrician has determined that your child is overweight:

- **Involve the entire family in healthier eating.** Do not single out your child as having a weight problem and as the only family member who cannot ever have treats.

- **Limit excess calories** by avoiding certain higher-calorie foods that offer little or no nutritional value, such as sugary carbonated soft drinks and juice beverages, cookies, and chips.

- **Focus on your child's health and positive qualities**, not her weight.

- **Walk the walk.** You're in this as a family, so be a positive role model for your child. If your son or daughter sees you eating breakfast, drinking low-fat milk, enjoying family meals, and getting regular physical activity, he or she is more likely to follow suit, now and for the rest of their lives.

- **Eat together as often as possible.** Family meals tend to include more whole grains, fruits, vegetables, low-fat (1%) milk, and fewer sugary beverages. Dining together also offers the opportunity to bond with your children.

Overfed and Undernourished

Many American children consume too many calories and too few nutrients. Like their adult counterparts, children often come up short for calcium, vitamin D, potassium, and dietary fiber. Overweight or not, a constant shortfall of these nutrients sets kids up for chronic conditions, including high blood pressure and osteoporosis, down the road.

Kids get about 35% of their calories from added solid fats (including butter, lard, stick margarine, shortening, and the fat in whole milk and fatty meats) and added sugars. In addition, children consume far more sodium, and far fewer whole grains than MyPlate and the 2010 Dietary Guidelines recommend. It's no wonder when you see the top calorie contributors (below, in descending order) in the daily diets of American children ages two to 18 years:

1. Grain-based desserts, including cake, cookies, pie, cobbler, sweet rolls, pastries, and donuts
2. Pizza
3. Yeast breads, including white bread or rolls, mixed-grain bread, flavored bread, whole-wheat bread, and bagels
4. Chicken and mixed dishes with chicken including fried or baked chicken parts and chicken strips/patties, chicken stir-fries, chicken casseroles, chicken sandwiches, chicken salads, stewed chicken, and other chicken mixed dishes
5. Pasta and pasta dishes including macaroni and cheese, spaghetti, other pasta with or without sauces, lasagna, ravioli, and noodles

While many of these foods, including whole-wheat bread, stewed chicken, and noodles, are healthy in their own right, American children clearly favor refined carbohydrates and processed foods with added solid fats, sodium, and sugar. For example, a cup of cooked pasta tossed with 2 teaspoon of a healthy trans-fat free tub spread, such as I Can't Believe It's Not Butter!®, and 1 teaspoon grated Parmesan cheese has about 300 calories and about 75 milligrams of sodium. While a cup of the same amount of macaroni and cheese prepared from a box supplies slightly fewer calories (260), it has nearly eight times the sodium (580 milligrams).

Closing Nutrient Gaps

Using MyPlate as a pattern for better eating helps to fill in the gaps in kids' diets (and those of adults) while promoting calorie balance. Make these six small changes to boost nutrition and keep calories in check.

1. Eat more whole grains, fruits, and vegetables. Pile half of MyPlate with fruits and vegetables, and about half of it with whole grains. Whole grains and produce are filling and they provide dietary fiber and potassium. Fruits and vegetables are loaded with water and dietary fiber, and such foods tend to have relatively fewer calories for the nutrients they supply.

In the Drink

Children ages two to 18 years average 400 calories from beverages every day. When they are young, most of these liquid calories come from milk and 100% juice. As they get older, taste preferences gravitate toward sugary carbonated soft drinks, sports drinks, and energy beverages. As a result, preteens and teens drink less milk, which is rich in several nutrients vital for growth, including calcium and vitamin D.

2. Reduce sugar-sweetened drinks. MyPlate recommends between two and three servings of fat-free and low-fat (1%) dairy, including milk and yogurt, every day. Older children and teens who drink more sugary beverages, such as juice drinks, sports drinks, and carbonated soft drinks often have higher body weight as compared to those who drink less. With the exception of flavored milk, sweetened beverages offer little in the way of nutrition. Offer children water, or fat-free or low-fat (1%) milk instead.

3. Get kids moving. Children who are physically active on a regular basis are stronger than children who are not. They also typically have less body fat and stronger bones, and they may experience reduced symptoms of anxiety and depression, according to the 2008 Physical Activity Guidelines for Americans.

Active kids also have a better chance of becoming healthier adults. Younger children, ages two to five, should play actively several times each day. Kids ages six to 17 years need 60 minutes or more of daily physical activity, most of it as aerobic activity of either moderate- or vigorous-intensity, and should include vigorous-intensity activity at least three times a week. As part of their 60 minutes or more, children and teens should include a muscle-strengthening activity on at least three days of the week, and activities that strengthen their bones, too, including walking, running, climbing, and, for older kids, resistance training.

4. Pull the plug. Time spent in front of a TV or computer screen means less time spent in physical activity. It may also be associated with overeating high-fat foods. A 2011 Harvard School of Public Health study found watching television is linked to greater weight gain over time. The American Academy of Pediatrics recommends no television for children ages two and under. Older children should restrict screen time to under two hours a day of quality programming.

5. Serve up a balanced breakfast. The State of the Family Nutrition and Physical Activity, a 2010 report from the American Dietetic Association (ADA) and the ADA Foundation, suggests that breakfast is the meal kids miss most often. Breakfast is an opportunity for good nutrition, and can help children include calcium, vitamin D, fiber, and potassium in their diet. In addition, children and teens who are regular breakfast eaters typically have a lower risk for being overweight. The morning meal also prevents hunger that saps a child's energy to learn and play.

Children and teens who are regular breakfast eaters typically have a lower risk for being overweight. What's more, the morning meal prevents hunger that saps a child's energy to learn and play.

The best breakfasts—including whole-grain cereal, fat-free or low-fat (1%) milk, and fruit—offer nutritious foods from at least three food groups, along with adequate protein. Protein helps to keep kids fuller longer, and protein-packed foods—such as milk, yogurt, and eggs—also supply the vitamins and minerals kids need to grow. Don't worry if your child doesn't like traditional breakfast foods. There are plenty of MyPlate combinations in the following list to entice your child to the table in the morning, or help him to include breakfast while on the run.

- Frozen whole-grain waffle sandwich with sunflower seed butter, peanut or almond butter, California raisins, and low-fat yogurt
- Vanilla-Mango Parfait: Layer low-fat lemon or vanilla yogurt with sliced fresh or previously frozen mango and crunchy whole-grain cereal in a glass or in an ice cream cone to take on the go.
- Hot cocoa (made with milk) or chocolate milk, slice of whole-grain toast, and fruit

- Breakfast Berry Parfait: Layer low-fat cottage cheese with whole-grain cereal and fresh or frozen berries
- Hard-cooked egg, such as Eggland's Best®, (make 6 or so on the weekend), fruit, and ½ whole-wheat English muffin with trans-fat free tub margarine (Choose a healthy spread made without hydrogenated oil and with no trans fat listed on the Nutrient Facts panel, such as I Can't Believe It's Not Butter!®, Country Crock®, and Promise Buttery Spread®.)
- Banana smoothie: Blend 1 cup low-fat (1%) milk with a medium banana and 1 teaspoon vanilla extract in a blender or food processor. Serve with ½ whole-wheat English muffin topped with trans-fat free tub margarine.
- Slice of pizza and 100% orange juice with calcium and vitamin D
- Turkey or roast beef roll up with cheese on a whole-wheat wrap
- Whole-grain roll, 1½ ounces hard cheese, such as cheddar, and sliced pear
- Half of a sandwich, milk, and fruit
- Sliced cheddar cheese melted on top of whole-wheat tortilla and low-sodium vegetable juice
- Whole-wheat graham crackers, hard-cooked egg, and a small banana
- Mini-pizza: Layer a small whole-wheat pita round with marinara sauce and grated reduced-fat cheddar cheese. Toast or broil.
- Whole-wheat bagel (mini for younger kids) spread with sunflower seed butter, almond butter, or peanut butter and drizzled with honey; 100% orange juice with calcium and vitamin D
- Plain low-fat yogurt topped with chopped walnuts, California raisins, and molasses or honey
- Plain, 1-minute or instant oatmeal microwaved with low-fat (1%) milk and topped with ¼ cup dried fruit and 2 tablespoons chopped almonds

6. Snack smart. Most kids need to snack, but many are snacking far too often.

Children eat 168 more calories as snacks every day than they did in 1977, an amount equal to the calories in 17 pounds of body fat.

There's nothing wrong with snacking. Problem is, snacks are often synonymous with highly processed foods rich in added sugar, fat, and sodium, including orange crackers, chips, cookies, and candy. Such foods nearly always lack the nutrients kids require, too.

When it comes to snacking, an attitude adjustment may be in order. Start thinking of snacks as mini-meals, and they won't be meal-wreckers. Offer children the same types of foods you would at any healthy meal, such as low-fat (1%) dairy and other lean protein sources, eggs, whole grains, fruits, and vegetables.

Snacks should combine protein and carbohydrate, at the very least. Fiber-rich foods (which contain carbohydrate) and protein help to keep kids fuller for longer. In addition, these foods tend to be rich in nutrients, too.

Here are some smart snack choices:

- Hummus, guacamole (look for the 100-calorie packs in the refrigerator section), or a small can of bean dip with baked snack chips or toasted whole-wheat pita bread, broken into chips
- Low-fat microwave popcorn tossed with Parmesan cheese
- Trail mix: Combine ½ cup of whole-grain cereal, ¼ cup California raisins or dried cranberries and 2 tablespoons each of sunflower seeds or chopped nuts, such as almonds, pecans, or walnuts. This is a good breakfast choice when served with a cup of low-fat (1%) milk or low-fat yogurt.
- Low-fat ice cream topped with fresh fruit
- Snack size (8 ounce) box of low-fat plain or chocolate milk and whole-wheat pretzels
- Whole-grain crackers, string cheese, such as Sargento Reduced Sodium String Cheese®, and dried figs
- Cooked or raw vegetables with low-fat Ranch dressing, and a hard-cooked egg
- Instant oatmeal made with milk in the microwave with 1 teaspoon cocoa powder stirred in and topped with sliced raspberries or strawberries
- Whole-wheat pretzels with peanut butter, almond butter, or sunflower seed butter
- Bowl of cereal and low-fat (1%) or fat-free milk
- Edamame
- Small container Greek yogurt
- Mini bagel spread with low-fat cream cheese and strawberry jam, and low-fat (1%) or fat-free milk

- Half a sandwich and glass of 100% orange juice with calcium and vitamin D
- Slice of pizza
- Hard-cooked egg and whole-grain roll
- Pistachios in the shell and glass of chocolate milk

Mom, Your Child's Health Is In Your Hands

You may be able to head off childhood obesity at the pass, well before your baby is born. After all, the womb is a child's first environment, and scientific research shows that the nine months spent there can shape his chances for a healthy weight years down the road.

If you're thinking about starting a family, or adding to yours, it's important to consider that your pre-pregnancy weight is a powerful weapon in the battle of the bulge. According to the 2010 Dietary Guidelines, women in their childbearing years who may become pregnant should try to keep their weight within a healthy range.

Starting pregnancy at a healthy weight, and gaining the recommended pregnancy pounds, helps to "program" your child against becoming overweight as a child. In addition, when you gain the amount of weight that's right for you during pregnancy, you reduce the risk for pregnancy complications, and you have an easier time of shedding baby weight, which improves your health and well-being in the long run.

Starting pregnancy at a healthy weight, and gaining the recommended pregnancy pounds, helps to "program" your child against becoming overweight as a child.

Women who are already pregnant and overweight should not put themselves on a weight-loss diet. Discuss your pregnancy weight gain with your doctor and consult with a registered dietitian (R.D.) to design an eating plan that works for you.

Perhaps you're not ready for pregnancy yet. Nevertheless, it pays to stay in shape, as nearly half of the pregnancies in the U.S. are unexpected or mistimed.

What's the right pregnancy weight gain for you?

Guidelines released in 2009 by the Institute of Medicine (IOM) suggest that your pre-pregnancy body mass index (BMI) determines the amount of recommended weight for pregnancy, along with the number of children you're carrying.

Gaining the suggested amount of weight based on your pre-pregnancy BMI reduces the risk of pre-term birth (delivery before 37 weeks) and promotes a baby that's neither too big nor too small.

What if your pregnancy weight gain isn't within the recommended range? Chances are, it won't make much of a difference if you're off by just a few pounds either way. The IOM guidelines provide a range in each BMI category, highlighting the fact that positive pregnancy outcomes are possible with different weight gains.

Refer to the chart on page 4 to determine your pre-pregnancy BMI, and use it as a starting point for pregnancy weight gain.

Here is a summary of weight gain guidelines for a single baby:

If Your BMI Is:	Your Total Weight Gain Should Be:
Less than 18.5	28 to 40 pounds
18.5 to 24.9	25 to 35 pounds
25 to 29.9	15 to 25 pounds
30 or greater	11 to 20 pounds

For twins:

If Your BMI Is:	Your Total Weight Gain Should Be:
Less than 18.5	Ask your doctor
18.5 to 24.9	37 to 54 pounds
25 to 29.9	31 to 50 pounds
30 or greater	25 to 42 pounds

Source: Institute of Medicine, 2009

Important Nutrients for Women

In addition to being mindful about their weight, the 2010 Dietary Guidelines advise future moms and pregnant women about two important nutrients—folic acid and iron—that are necessary to help their babies grow and develop to their fullest potential.

Folic Acid

Women capable of becoming pregnant need: 400 micrograms (mcg) of folic acid every day, in addition to foods rich in folate, such as orange juice, dark green leafy vegetables, lentils, and strawberries.

Pregnant women need: 600 mcg of folic acid daily, in addition to folate-rich foods.

About folic acid: Folic acid, a B-vitamin, is the synthetic form of folate, which is found naturally in certain plant foods. During the first month of pregnancy, folic acid and folate help to head off certain birth defects, including spina bifida. As pregnancy progresses, your baby needs folic acid and folate to grow and develop normally, and folate is necessary to reduce the risk of preterm birth.

Grains, including breakfast cereals, bread, pasta, and rice are typically fortified with folic acid, the same form of the vitamin that appears in dietary supplements. The Dietary Guidelines advise getting the folic acid you need from dietary supplements (over-the-counter multivitamins typically provide 400 mcg per pill) and/or fortified foods, in addition to eating a diet rich in folate-filled foods. It's not always easy to determine how much folic acid is found in a serving of fortified foods, so here's a guide:

Folate-Rich Food	Folate/ Folic Acid (mcg)
Breakfast cereals, fortified with 100% of Daily Value for folate, ¾ cup*	400
Asparagus, cooked, 8 spears	190
Spinach, frozen, cooked, 1 cup	100
Broccoli, chopped, frozen, cooked, 4 spears (5 inches long)	100
Rice, white, enriched, cooked, 1 cup*	130
White beans, canned, drained, ½ cup	123
Spaghetti, enriched, cooked, 1 cup*	92
Orange juice, fresh, 1 cup	74
Spinach, raw, 1 cup	60
Green peas, frozen, cooked, ½ cup	50
Strawberries, sliced, 1 cup	40

Source is added folic acid.
Source: Adapted from Dietary Supplement Fact Sheet: Folate.
http://ods.od.nih.gov/factsheets/Folate-HealthProfessional; USDA

Iron

Women capable of becoming pregnant need: Foods rich in heme iron as part of a balanced diet for a total of 18 milligrams (mg) a day.

Pregnant women need: Twenty seven milligrams a day, which can usually be achieved by taking a multivitamin and eating a balanced diet that includes iron-rich foods. It's important to get the iron you need every day, or risk deficiency.

About iron: Iron helps your body make hemoglobin, the part of red blood cells that transports oxygen to cells, among other functions.

Women who are capable of becoming pregnant, and pregnant women, should choose foods that supply *heme* iron on a regular basis. *Heme* iron is the primary form of iron found in animal foods, such as meat, seafood, and poultry. *Heme* iron is more readily absorbed by the body than *non-heme* iron, which is the only form of iron in plant foods, and in fortified products, such as bread, breakfast cereal, pasta, and rice. Pair vitamin C- rich choices such as orange juice, strawberries, tomato, and kiwi, and foods with *non-heme* iron to enhance the absorption of *non-heme* iron.

Iron-Rich Food	Iron (mg)
Oatmeal, fortified, instant, 1 packet*	11
Ready-to-eat breakfast cereal, ¾ to 1 cup*	10 to 22
Spinach, cooked, 1 cup*	6
Soybeans, cooked, ½ cup*	4
Rice, medium-grain, fortified, cooked, ½ cup*	4
Oysters, fried, 3½ ounces	3
Lentils, cooked, ½ cup*	3
Beef, ground, cooked, 3½ ounces	3
Turkey, dark meat, cooked, 3½ ounces	2
Chicken breast, skinless, cooked, 3½ ounces	1
Pork tenderloin, cooked, 3½ ounces	1

Contains added non-heme or naturally-occuring non-heme iron.
Source: USDA

Is Fish Safe to Eat While Pregnant?

In a first, the 2010 Dietary Guidelines call out seafood, giving it special significance among protein sources. They advise adults to eat at least eight ounces of seafood every week; pregnant and breastfeeding women should include eight to 12 ounces a week.

Scientific evidence suggests that the omega-3 fats, particularly docosahexaenoic acid (DHA), a healthy fat found in seafood, contributes to improved vision and brain function in babies during pregnancy and infancy.

Some seafood is safer than others, however. Women who are in their childbearing years should avoid shark, swordfish, tilefish, and king mackerel because of the potential for high mercury levels in these fish. Mercury is capable of damaging your child's developing brain and neurological system. (See pages 93-96 for more about the benefits of eating seafood and seafood safety.)

Eat Better At Home

Fast food, busy schedules, homework, large portions of relatively inexpensive foods such as chicken nuggets, French fries, and soft drinks are among the factors that conspire against us as we try to feed our children healthier fare. Since fast food places, giant chocolate chip cookies, and a hectic lifestyle aren't going away any time soon, you need to take the bull by the horns at home.

Being a parent doesn't mean you have perfect eating and exercise habits, but it won't hurt to try to be the best role model possible for your children, including when you're pregnant. You may think that children are not paying attention to how you live your life, but kids take their cues about the value of a balanced diet and regular physical activity from the adults around them. If you eat better and exercise more, chances are your child will, too. You won't always get it right every day, but at least you'll be trying to do better.

If you eat better and exercise more, chances are your child will, too. You won't always get it right every day, but at least you'll be trying to do better.

It's not easy to make changes at home, but it's well worth the effort. Children, even seemingly intractable teens, are highly suggestible, and they can learn to favor nutritious foods and regular physical activity. Find out more about how much exercise children need every day, and the benefits of physical activity for the entire family, in chapter three.

CHAPTER 3

Physical Activity on Your Plate

YOU DON'T SEE ANY FIGURES RUNNING CIRCLES around the MyPlate icon, but intuition tells you that physical activity is part of the MyPlate program. You're right.

Calorie intake matters when it comes to good health, but the energy adults and children consume is just one piece of the weight control equation. Physical activity balances calorie intake. Being physically active is one of the most important steps that nearly every American can take to improve their health, no matter what their age or weight. Everyone benefits from physical activity, including healthy people, those at risk for chronic conditions, such as heart disease and high blood pressure, people with physical disabilities, and children.

Physical activity balances calorie intake. Being physically active is one of the most important steps that nearly every American can take to improve their health, no matter what their age or weight.

The human body is meant to move, not to sit for as much as we do every day. The best way to be physically active is to take part in enjoyable activities that suit your stage of life. For children, playing, climbing, and running are natural movements that help them to grow and develop. Adults may need to alter their routines to compensate for time constraints, age, and injury. Even healthy pregnant women can work out until the day they deliver.

Moving around more offers a multitude of benefits that go beyond looking good in your jeans. As you read on, you'll find it difficult to argue with the confirmed benefits of physical activity. You may need some convincing to get a move on, or perhaps you just need some tips to incorporate more activity into your busy life. By the end of this chapter, even confirmed couch potatoes will have discovered at least one reason to get moving on a regular basis, and how best to get going.

The Difference Between Physical Activity and Exercise

Any activity is beneficial, and moving around more encourages the idea that physical activity is the norm in your life, and your family's, not the exception. But let's face it: some moves are better than others. All exercise is physical activity, but not all physical activity is exercise.

Exercise is a form of physical activity that is planned, structured, repetitive, and performed with the goal of improving health or fitness. When added to your baseline movement, exercise, such as brisk walking, jumping rope, dancing, lifting weights, and yoga, is beneficial.

That doesn't mean to discourage physical activity. The more active you are, the better, generally speaking. Doing anything, even for a short period of time, helps you to work up to getting the health-enhancing physical activity you need. Doing even moderate physical activity also helps older people and those whose movement may be limited for any reason. Even low levels of activity, like getting out of the car instead of using the drive-thru, taking the groceries in from the car one bag at a time, and getting up off the couch to change the TV channel, are preferable to an inactive lifestyle.

Why Physical Activity Matters

According to the 2008 Physical Activity Guidelines for Americans (PAG), only a few lifestyle choices are as beneficial to your health as regular physical activity.

People who are physically active for seven hours or more a week have a 40% lower risk of dying early than those who are active for less than 30 minutes a week. You're thinking: seven hours a week? That's not for me. The good news is that it's not necessary to perform hours and hours of physical activity for better health. Getting 150 minutes of moderate-intensity aerobic physical activity a week (30 minutes on most days of the week) will help you to live longer, and better, too.

Here are some of the many health benefits linked to regular physical activity:
- Burns calories, and, when balanced with calorie intake, helps prevent weight gain and helps with weight loss
- Curbs colon cancer risk
- Reduces the chances for breast cancer

- Reduces your risk for heart disease, stroke, some cancers, and osteoporosis
- Reduces the chances for developing type 2 diabetes and helps control blood glucose levels in people who have type 2 diabetes
- Reduces depression and improves brain function
- Lowers your chances of developing high blood pressure and elevated blood cholesterol levels, two risk factors for heart disease
- Lowers the risk of metabolic syndrome. Metabolic syndrome is a condition in which people have some combination of the following: high blood pressure, excess abdominal fat, low levels of high density lipoprotein (HDL or good cholesterol), high levels of triglycerides (fat) in the blood, and trouble keeping blood glucose levels within the normal range. Metabolic syndrome is a risk factor for cardiovascular disease.
- Strengthens your heart, lungs, and muscles
- Preserves and builds muscle, which may improve your calorie-burning capacity
- Helps prevent falls

What Type and How Much Physical Activity You Need

The PAG recommends combining different types of exercise to reap the most benefits.

Aerobic Activity

Aerobic activity is the type of physical activity that causes your heart to beat faster. It uses large muscle groups, like your legs, for a more sustained period of time. Aerobic means "with air." Aerobic activities are repetitive and require large amounts of oxygen to keep going. They include riding a bike, brisk walking, running, and swimming. Aerobic activity has three components:

- *Intensity*, which is how hard you work to do the activity. Walking

☐ Exercise, and keep cancer at bay?

Studies suggest a link between years of getting regular physical activity and a lower risk for certain cancers, especially breast cancer and colon cancer. It takes more than the recommended amount of exercise for the general public to thwart breast and colon cancer—between three and a half and seven hours a week of physical activity to confer some protection. That's about 40 minutes of exercise on five days a week to an hour, seven days a week. The evidence connecting exercise and endometrial cancer is not as strong as that for breast and colon cancer. However, some research suggests that the risk of endometrial cancer in women and lung cancer in men and women may be lower among those who are regularly active compared to inactive people.

and running are both aerobic activities, but running is more intense.

- *Frequency*, which is how often you do the activity.
- *Duration*, which is how long you do the activity.

The PAG factors intensity, frequency, and duration into the recommendations for how much exercise you need. Guidelines for adults focus on moderate-intensity activity and vigorous-intensity activity. You can do one or the other type of aerobic exercise or a combination of both to meet your exercise quota.

How can you tell if your activity is of moderate intensity? Generally speaking, you'll be able to talk, but not sing during the activity. You won't be able to say more than a few words without pausing for a breath during vigorous-intensity activities.

Choosing vigorous-intensity exercise can save time. That's because one minute of vigorous-intensity exercise equals two minutes of moderate-intensity activity. For example, 30 minutes of brisk walking (3 miles an hour at least) is roughly the same in terms of health benefits as running for 15 minutes.

Examples of moderate-intensity aerobic activities

- Walking briskly (3 miles an hour—20 minutes per mile—or faster, but not race-walking)
- Water aerobics
- Bicycling slower than 10 miles an hour (6 minutes per mile pace)
- Tennis (doubles)
- Ballroom and line dancing
- General gardening (raking, trimming shrubs, mowing the lawn)
- Downhill skiing
- Swimming
- Using hand cyclers—also known as ergometers
- Canoeing
- Sports where you catch and throw (baseball, softball, volleyball)
- Using your manual wheelchair

Examples of vigorous-intensity aerobic activities

- Racewalking, jogging, or running
- Swimming laps
- Basketball
- Ice or field hockey

- Vigorous dancing
- Soccer
- Martial arts (such as karate)
- Tennis (singles)
- Aerobic dancing
- Bicylcing 10 miles an hour—6 minutes per mile—or faster
- Jumping rope
- Heavy gardening (continuous digging or hoeing, with heart rate increases)
- Hiking uphill or with a heavy backpack
- Cross-country skiing
- Skateboarding and rollerblading

Frequency and Duration

As little as 60 minutes of physical activity a week will get you some health benefits, but you can reap substantial gains with a minimum of 2 hours and 30 minutes (at least 150 minutes or 30 minutes a day on most days of the week) of moderate-intensity physical activity or its equivalent as vigorous-intensity exercise a week.

You'll gain more extensive health and fitness benefits as you move toward 300 minutes (5 hours) weekly. Additional benefits include a lower risk of colon cancer and breast cancer and prevention of unhealthy weight gain as well as more reduced risk of heart disease or diabetes than someone who works out for 150 minutes a week.

Work Out At Work

Some people with active jobs, such as construction workers and postal carriers, may get enough on-the-job physical activity to meet the 2008 Physical Activity Guidelines for Americans.

Accumulate Your Exercise

You may have been operating under the assumption that it's best to get 30 minutes of exercise on five or more days a week. That's a fine approach, but the recommendation for accumulating exercise has been tweaked a bit in the 2008 PAG, and it's actually more accommodating for people with busy schedules.

Since it's not yet scientifically possible to determine whether the health benefits of 30 minutes on five days a week is any different from the health benefits of 50 minutes on three days a week, the latest exercise guidelines say that *accumulating 150 minutes a week should be the focus.*

That's great news for people who are strapped for time and can't fit in exercise every day. Do try to spread exercise over three days during the week to reduce injury risk and prevent excessive fatigue.

Muscle-Strengthening Activity

Muscle-strengthening activity works the muscles by causing them to hold against an applied force or weight, which could be a hand-held dumbbell, elastic bands, weight machines, or your own body weight.

Muscle-strengthening activities, such as weight training, rock climbing, and push ups, exhaust the smaller muscle groups.

Muscle-strengthening activities have three components.

- *Intensity*, which is how much weight or force is used.
- *Frequency*, which is how often a person does the activity.
- *Repetitions*, which is how many times you lift a weight, do a push up, or complete a chin-up.

Because the effects of muscle-strengthening activities are limited to the muscle groups being worked, it's important to target all the major muscle groups, including the legs, hips, back, belly, chest, shoulders, and arms, on a regular basis.

Because the effects of muscle-strengthening activities are limited to the muscle groups being worked, it's important to target all the major muscle groups, including the legs, hips, back, belly, chest, shoulders, and arms, on a regular basis. Muscle-strengthening activities for all the major muscle groups should be done at least twice a week on two different days. In addition to the more obvious types of muscle-strengthening activity—such as weight training and working out with resistance bands—carrying heavy loads, and gardening that includes hoeing and digging qualify, too.

There's no time recommendation on strength-training activities, but you should do them to the point at which you can't do anymore. In resistance training, one set of eight to 12 repetitions of each exercise is effective.

Bone-Strengthening Activity

Bone-strengthening activities promote bone growth and bone strength by exerting force on the skeleton. Activities that strengthen muscles, including weight training, may also boost bone strength. Many aerobic activities, including brisk walking, jumping jacks, and running, also serve to bolster bone strength. Bone-strengthening activities can be aerobic or muscle strengthening, or both, such as jumping jacks.

☐ Any Movement Matters

The adult physical activity guidelines in the 2008 PAG are intended for people ages 18 to 64. Adults ages 65 and older should follow the adult guidelines. If you're over 65 and you can't meet the minimum suggested amount of daily exercise, do what you can, and be as active as your physical abilities and medical conditions allow. Remember, any movement is beneficial. Generally speaking, the more you move around, the more you are able to move around.

Get Motivated to Move

Increasing your physical activity level can be daunting, especially if you think you must hit the 150-minute mark during your first week! If you've been inactive, you can easily become overwhelmed by that goal. Try not to let it get the better of your motivation to move around more. Instead, work gradually toward the goal.

When you start, spread your sessions throughout the week and make activity light to moderate in intensity. There is no reason to rush; you'll get there! If you become frustrated, just remember that any activity is better than none, and that, just by moving for a few minutes at a time, you are making progress.

You don't have to join a gym or pay for a personal trainer to make strides to better health. Walking, even for an extra 10 minutes a day, is a great way to increase your physical activity level. Don't forget to include muscle-strengthening activities. Aim for one day a week at a light or moderate level, then work up to at least two times weekly, and increase the intensity until it becomes moderate to high. Use free weights or resistance bands at home or follow along with your favorite TV exercise show.

If you have a medical condition, get the green light from your physician before you begin any exercise routine.

Putting Together a Plan for Physical Activity

Here are some examples of how to get the equivalent of 150 minutes of moderate-intensity and muscle-strengthening activities the PAG recommends every week:

- 30 minutes of walking for five days + two days of resistance bands
- 25 minutes of running on three days + lifting weights on 2 days
- 30 minutes of brisk walking on 2 days + 60 minutes of dancing + 30 minutes of mowing the lawn + heavy gardening on 2 days
- 60 minutes of aerobic dance class + 30 minutes of brisk walking + boot camp-style class (push ups, calisthenics, etc.) on 3 different days
- 30 minutes of biking to and from work on 3 days + playing softball for 60 minutes + using weight machines or free weights on 2 different days
- 45 minutes of brisk doubles tennis on 2 days + lifting weights on 1 day + hiking for 30 minutes and rock climbing

If you do even more than 150 minutes a week of moderate-intensity physical activity, use these suggestions to boost your activity.

- 45 minutes of brisk walking every day + exercising with resistance bands on 2 or 3 days
- 45 minutes of running on 3 to 4 days + circuit weight training in a gym on 2 or 3 days
- 30 minutes of running on 2 days; 45 minutes of brisk walking + 45 minutes of aerobic and weights class + 90 minutes of dancing + 30 minutes of mowing the lawn + heavy garden work
- 90 minutes of basketball + brisk walking for 15 minutes on 3 days + lifting weights on 2 days
- 45 minutes of stationary bicycling on 2 days + 60 minutes of soccer on 2 days + calisthenics on 3 days

Keep Kids Active

Children are naturally active, but as they get older, they spend more time sitting—in school, in front of TV and computer screens, doing homework, and communicating with their friends through electronic devices. Helping children to make physical activity the rule, and not the exception, lays the foundation for a healthier life by setting a strong example early on.

Teens and younger children who get regular physical activity have stronger hearts, lungs, bones, and muscles. Generally speaking, active children are also leaner, and they may experience fewer symptoms of anxiety and depression.

Regular physical activity beginning early in life reduces the chances that children will develop risk factors, including high blood pressure, excess weight and obesity, and elevated blood cholesterol levels, that contribute to so-called "adult diseases" such as heart disease and type 2 diabetes.

Like adults, children between the ages of six and 17 require a combination of aerobic and muscle-strengthening activities. Bone strengthening activities, including running, jumping, basketball, gymnastics, volleyball, and tennis, are also important, and can be either aerobic activities or muscle-strengthening activities.

It's important to remember that kids, especially younger ones, are active in a more intermittent way than adults. Children tend to alternate brief periods of aerobic activity, such as running, skipping, and jumping, with brief periods of rest. That's different from how most adults get their activity, which is often as a 30-minute walk, biking for an hour, or swimming laps for 20 minutes. Another difference: Younger kids don't typically require a formal muscle-strengthening program, like weight-lifting, to build muscle strength. They often use unstructured play, such as climbing, swinging on playground equipment/bars, and playing tug-of-war to get stronger.

Kids can meet their physical-activity needs with a combination of moderate- and vigorous-intensity activity to help improve their heart and lung strength.

Kids can meet their physical-activity needs with a combination of moderate- and vigorous-intensity activity to help improve their heart and lung strength. A brisk walk to school is an activity with moderate intensity, while running on the playground is considered vigorous. Children should always engage in activities that are safe and appropriate for their age.

How much exercise for your child?

The following PAG guidelines are for children ages six to 17.

- 60 minutes or more of physical activity daily, most of it as aerobic activity of either moderate- or vigorous-intensity, and should include vigorous-intensity activity at least three times a week.
- As part of their 60 minutes or more of daily physical activity, children and teens should include muscle-strengthening activity on at least three days of the week.

◻ Kids Need to Move It

When it comes to physical activity, American kids are all over the map. Some don't come close to satisfying the guidelines, while others exceed them. Inactive kids should gradually increase their activity levels doing activities they enjoy. Children who meet the guidelines should, if they can, become even more physically active. Those who exceed the PAG guidelines should keep up the good work and vary the kinds of activities they do to reduce the risk of injury.

- As part of their 60 minutes or more of daily physical activity, children and teens should include bone-strengthening physical activity on at least three days of the week.

Family Fitness and Fun

Physical activity is a way to have fun, spend time with family and friends, enjoy the outdoors in all seasons, and improve fitness.

- **Walk, bike, or jog together** on a regular basis, before or after dinner on most nights of the week.
- **Work with your kids to develop a list** of regular activities you can do together, rain or shine, such as mall walking, playing basketball at the Y or other gym, swimming at an indoor pool, and tennis.
- **Take an exercise class together,** such as yoga or kick-boxing, through community education programs or park and recreation programs.
- **Choose an active vacation,** where lots of walking, biking, hiking, or water sports are readily available.
- **Plan active birthday parties,** such as playing laser tag, rock climbing, and swimming.
- **When the weather is bad, rely on active video games** and DVDs to get moving or follow along with a free exercise show on TV.
- **Train for an event with your kids,** such as a charity walk, run, or bike race.
- **Toss or kick a ball in the backyard,** or play Frisbee or tag with your kids. Fly a kite at the beach or in a park.
- **See who can take the most steps.** Buy everyone in the family pedometers and compete to see who moves more. Keep a chart and tally steps at the end of the week.
- **Be prepared.** Have family members stash sports equipment, like sneakers, basketballs, soccer balls, and tennis racquets in the car. That way, you're always ready to include physical activity when the opportunity arises.

Exercise: Work It In

There is a laundry list of reasons to exercise, and one that is nearly as long for why people don't work out. Given the multitude of health benefits exercise provides, it's surprising to note that only one in three Americans gets the recommended amount of activity.

What are your barriers? Perhaps you lack the time to exercise or you think it's inconvenient because you're busy or you travel a lot. Maybe you think working out is a bore.

Everyone, even the most dedicated of exercisers, loses their motivation to work out from time to time. Chances are, your physical activity and exercise routine will change as time goes on, creating obstacles to exercise. Pregnancy, parenthood, age, illness, injury, reduced energy level, and any other change in your lifestyle can put a crimp in the amount of time and energy you have for working out. There's almost always a solution to the one, or more, obstacles that prevent you from getting the exercise you need.

Can't Get to the Gym?

Work out at home. It may not be the most ideal situation for you, but it's better than nothing. Take a walk or run, starting from your house. Have a set of weights and bands and DVDs or shows available to follow along with. If you're going to be nearly housebound for a while, like right after delivering a baby, invest in a treadmill or elliptical machine for aerobic workouts, if you can afford it.

Are You Bored?

Choose activities you enjoy. People who are regular exercisers should add variety to their workouts to prevent boredom. For example, if you run five days a week, cut back to three and add an aerobic activity such as kick-boxing classes, Zumba®, or swimming two times weekly. In addition to working your muscles in a different way, variety is helpful for reducing the risk of injury caused by doing too much of any one activity.

Do You Need More of a Challenge?

Experienced walkers or runners can up the ante by adding hills to their course or running the same course in the reverse order to challenge muscles. Or, you can work out more, aiming for upwards of 300 minutes of moderate-intensity activity or 150 minutes of vigorous-intensity physical activity a week, more intense muscle-strengthening activity on at least two days a week, or both.

Do You Have a Busy Schedule?

Everyone should schedule working out and treat exercise like an important client, friend, or family member. Travelers should choose hotels with fitness centers or pools to get a work out in. Keeping a log of your exercise helps you to see how often you are physically active.

Do You Need Motivation?

If you lack get-up-and-go, enlist a friend or co-worker to work out with, join a walking group, or take an exercise class. Having others keep tabs on you makes it more difficult to skip days or cut corners. Exercise with a few friends, so if one can't make it, you always have someone to be active with.

Overcoming the Time Crunch

Pressed for time? Here are some 10-minute blocks of moderate-intensity and vigorous-intensity activities that you and your children can squeeze into your day to meet exercise goals.

- Park your car farther away from your work place or get off public transportation a few blocks farther away and sneak in a brisk walk to and from work every day.
- Bike to work or to do your errands.
- Walk the dog twice a day. Don't have a dog? Offer to walk someone else's.
- Pedal on a stationary bike or walk on a treadmill. Watch TV or listen to music to keep it interesting.
- Walk with a friend rather than lingering over coffee or a drink.
- Pace while waiting for elevators. Walk up and down the airport halls when waiting for your plane to board.

Pregnancy and Physical Activity: Yes, you can!

Regular physical activity during pregnancy helps you gain the right amount of weight, and so much more. Physical activity during pregnancy improves heart and lung strength and boosts your mood, and may reduce the risk of pregnancy complications, such as gestational diabetes. Exercise may even reduce the time it takes to deliver your baby.

Moderate-intensity physical activity is safe for healthy pregnant women, and experts recommend it highly. Even if you were relatively inactive before you conceived, you can begin to work up to the 150-minute-a-week goal. Women who are already that active can continue with their moderate-intensity aerobic physical activity during pregnancy and after delivery day, as long

◻ Stay on Track

You can keep tabs on your physical activity and gradually increase it to meet the recommendations of the 2008 Physical Activity Guidelines for Americans at www.presidentschallenge.org or with a log like this one found at www.health.gov/paguidelines.

as they check with their doctor first. Women with certain complications of pregnancy, including pregnancy-induced hypertension (high blood pressure) and pre-term labor are often advised to avoid physical activity. If you have these conditions, or any others, consult your doctor about how much activity is right for you.

If you're just beginning to get more physically active or if you're already active, ask your doctor or midwife about adjusting physical activity during pregnancy and after delivery. You may be more comfortable with programs that are tailored to your needs, such as yoga and strength-training classes for pregnant women. You'll tire more easily as the pregnancy progresses, so be aware that the aerobic activity you've been doing all along may be more of a challenge for you. Now is not the time to take up a strenuous sport.

If you're just beginning to get more physical activity or if you're already active, ask your doctor or midwife about adjusting physical activity during pregnancy and after delivery.

Women who regularly do vigorous activity or lots of strength training should continue with their routines, but pay attention to potential limits on their activity, especially as their due date approaches. Be sure to wear comfortable clothes and supportive sneakers, get plenty of fluid before, during, and after physical activity, and to work out in cool, well-ventilated places. Women who exercise regularly need to account for the calories they burn. This is especially true for women who were sedentary before conceiving a child, and who begin a regular physical activity routine during pregnancy.

Certain activities are off-limits during pregnancy, no matter how accomplished you are at them. Any activity that involves pressure changes or with a high risk of falling or abdominal injury are not considered safe for pregnant women. The following activities are out of the question during pregnancy:

- Surfing
- Kickboxing
- Downhill skiing or snowboarding
- Waterskiing
- Horseback riding
- Skateboarding
- Roller skating
- Ice skating
- Bike riding (stationary bike riding is OK)
- Contact sports, including ice hockey, soccer, touch or tackle football, lacrosse, and basketball
- Gymnastics
- Rock climbing
- Skydiving
- Anything with jumping or jarring motions

Slow Burn, All Day Long

While it's beneficial to get 30 or even 60 minutes of exercise every day, it's even better to move around as much as possible. The following list of everyday activities burn about 100 calories for a 150-pound person. People who weigh more will burn more, and vice versa.

Do this	For this many minutes
Walk up the stairs during the day	11
Kick a soccer ball with your kids	13
Shovel snow	15
Shoot hoops	20
Mow the lawn	20
Play golf (no cart)	20
Light yard work	20
Play tag with the kids	22
Ride a bike (about 10 miles per hour)	22
Wash the car	30
Bowling	30
Toss a ball with your kids	30

Adapted from Ainsworth, B., et al. "Compendium of Physical Activities: An Update of Activity Codes and MET Intensities." Medicine & Science in Sports and Exercise, 32 (9 Suppl): S498-504, 2000.

Make Your Move

You've probably guessed at the overriding idea in this chapter: Avoid inactivity at all costs. Lack of motivation, time, or energy—or all three—put a real, or imaginary crimp in regular exercise routines. Here's what matters most: do what you can to move around more, whenever you can, and to get the children in your life to do the same. Physical activity counts towards better health.

In the next chapter, you'll learn about how best to make your calories count, too.

CHAPTER 4

Make Calories Count

WHEN YOU LOOK AT MYPLATE, you see that it's not divided up into four equal portions representing the major food groups. Yet, it promotes a balanced diet, as long as you're not eating off a giant dinner plate, that is!

Eating and drinking more calories than you need upsets your personal calorie balance and leads to weight gain. Nobody ever became overweight eating carrot sticks and lettuce, however. Overindulging on foods that are loaded with added fats, sugar, and sodium, and low in fiber, makes it easier to pack on the pounds and hold onto extra weight.

To make matters worse, we're overfed and undernourished. The foods and beverages that we choose on a regular basis often fail to supply the vitamins, minerals, fiber, and other nutrients necessary for good health, now, and in the future. The same goes for our children, who are still developing and often have much higher nutrient needs than adults.

The good news is that, using MyPlate, you and your family can make simple changes to restore balance to your diet.

Calcium, vitamin D, potassium, and fiber are in particularly short supply for most adults and children, according to the 2010 Dietary Guidelines for Americans. The opposite is true for sodium, which many people eat in copious quantities. In addition, most men consume too much cholesterol, and some people drink more calories than they need in the form of alcoholic beverages.

The combination of extra calories and poor food choices has created a perfect storm for promoting heart disease, high blood pressure, type 2 diabetes, and certain cancers. That's the bad news. The good news is that, using MyPlate, you and your family can make simple changes to restore balance to your diet. Read on for a description of the nutrients you may be missing out on, and easy ways to work them into your family's eating plan.

Capitalize on Calcium

Your bones and teeth store about 99% of all the calcium in your body, but calcium does more than just bolster bone strength and thickness. The remaining 1%, found in the blood and tissues, perpetuates life by promoting normal muscle contraction, nerve transmission, and a regular heartbeat.

When your diet is low in calcium, your body "withdraws" the mineral from the skeleton to keep blood and tissue calcium concentrations within a healthy range. If your body takes more calcium from bones than it "deposits" from eating foods and taking dietary supplements, bones become progressively weaker and prone to breaking.

Daily calcium requirements differ with age and gender. During adolescence the body achieves peak bone mass, so getting enough calcium is especially important for pre-teens and teenagers. This may come as a surprise, but pregnancy and breastfeeding don't alter your daily calcium needs:

- One to three year-olds: 500 milligrams (mg)
- Four to eight year-olds: 800 mg
- Nine to 18 year-olds: 1,300 mg
- 19 to 50 year-olds: 1,000 mg (males)
- 50 years and older: 1,200 mg (females), 1,000 mg (males)

Source: Institute of Medicine, 2010

Calcium-Containing Foods

Dairy foods supply the greatest concentration of natural calcium, which is why they're considered excellent choices for fulfilling your daily calcium quota. Certain fish are reliable calcium sources, too. Fortified plant foods also help to fulfill calcium needs.

Food	Calcium (milligrams)
Yogurt, plain, non-fat, 1 cup	452
Yogurt, fruit-flavored, 1 cup	345
Swiss cheese, 1½ ounces	336
Cheddar cheese, 1½ ounces	307

Food	Calcium (milligrams)
Low-fat milk (1%) or fat-free milk, 8 ounces	300
Lactose-reduced milk, such as Lactaid®	300
Orange juice, calcium fortified, 8 ounces	300 - 500
Soy beverages, original and vanilla, calcium-fortified	299
Chocolate milk, low-fat (1%), 8 ounces	290
Salmon, pink, canned, 3½ ounces	263
Tofu, firm, prepared with calcium sulfate, ½ cup	204

Source: USDA

Vitamin D In Your Diet

Think of vitamin D as calcium's silent partner. Without vitamin D, the body has difficulty absorbing calcium from foods, beverages, and dietary supplements, and directing the flow of calcium in and out of bones.

Vitamin D's primary role is bolstering bone strength in children and adults, but emerging evidence from observational studies suggests it plays a part in preventing certain types of cancers, helps to head off cardiovascular disease, and prevents immune system disorders, including multiple sclerosis.

That's not all vitamin D does. It also influences cell growth and immune function, tamps down inflammation, and helps your nervous system to work properly. While vitamin D is being studied for its potential role in preventing and treating chronic conditions, to date, its best-known function is supporting bone health.

Vitamin D also influences cell growth and immune function, tamps down inflammation, and helps your nervous system to work properly.

Your body can make all the vitamin D it needs, as long as you have some "unprotected sun." You must expose your skin to strong summer sunshine to trigger vitamin D production in the skin. Many of us fail to make the vitamin D our body requires because we use sunscreens with a Sun Protection Factor (SPF) of 8 or above, avoid the sun, live in the northern part of the country where the sun is too weak to initiate vitamin D production for about half the year, or a combination of the above. Having dark skin or being overweight makes vitamin D deficiency more likely. People with a Body Mass Index (BMI) of ≥ 30 may need more vitamin D than those who weigh less to obtain optimal blood levels of vitamin D.

Breastfed babies need supplemental vitamin D. Human milk is relatively low in vitamin D, and infants who are exclusively breast-fed run a high risk of vitamin D deficiency. The American Academy of Pediatrics recommends that all breast-fed and partially breast-fed infants receive 400 International Units (IU) of supplemental vitamin D daily starting in the first days of life. Ask your pediatrician for guidance on vitamin D supplements.

Vitamin D-Rich Foods

Few foods naturally supply vitamin D. Fortified foods, including milk, eggs, and orange juice, help you to get the vitamin D you need. If you can't get enough vitamin D through food, use dietary supplements to fill the gap in your diet, and your child's.

Everyone ages one to 70 requires 600 IU of vitamin D daily. If you're older than 70, you need 800 IU a day. People over the age of nine should not consume more than 4,000 IU a day of vitamin D.

Food	Vitamin D (IU)
Salmon, sockeye, cooked, 3 ounces	447
Monterey Mushrooms (grown in UV* light), raw, 3 ounces	400
Tuna, light, canned in oil, drained, 3 ounces	216
Mushrooms, morel, raw, 3 ounces	173
Orange juice, vitamin D fortified, 8 ounces	136
Milk, all types, 8 ounces	116
Low-fat chocolate milk (1%), 8 ounces	112
Soy beverage, vitamin D fortified, 8 ounces	108
Cereal, ready-to-eat, fortified, ¾ to 1 cup	36-100
Eggland's Best egg, large, 1	80
Pork, various cuts, cooked, 3 ounces	24-88

* Ultraviolet light. Mushrooms naturally produce vitamin D after exposure to UV light.
Source: USDA

Pack in Potassium

The mineral potassium is part of every cell of your body. It plays a key role in fluid balance and keeping your brain, nerves, heart, and muscles functioning normally on a constant basis.

As part of a healthy diet, potassium counters the effects of sodium, which promotes water retention, and helps promote normal blood pressure. It also helps to head off bone loss and kidney stones. African Americans and people with high blood pressure especially benefit from consuming the suggested intake of potassium.

The 2010 Dietary Guidelines suggests 4,700 milligrams (mg) of potassium daily. When you think of potassium-rich foods, orange juice and bananas probably come to mind. In reality, potassium is found in substantial amounts in fresh and lightly processed foods, including dairy products. Eight ounces of low-fat chocolate milk packs as much potassium as a medium banana.

Processing and cooking reduce potassium levels. For example, one medium baked potato serves up nearly twice the potassium of the same amount of highly processed potato puffs. To get more potassium, eat foods that are as close to their original state as possible to maximize the mineral.

Food First, Then Supplements

Experts prefer you get the nutrients you need from foods. Nutrient-rich foods provide vitamins, minerals, and other beneficial compounds, such as fiber and phytonutrients found in plant foods, that supplements don't supply. However, dietary supplements and fortified foods may be necessary to supply vitamin D, folic acid, vitamin B12, and iron, according to the 2010 Dietary Guidelines. A regular multivitamin may be useful for filling in other, small nutrient gaps, too.

Mind Your Medications

Certain medications, such as diuretics to lower blood pressure, affect potassium requirements. Ask your doctor or pharmacist about how all of the medications you take affect the potassium levels in your body.

Potassium-Packed Foods

Food	Potassium (mg)
Potato, baked, with skin, medium	926
Yogurt, plain, fat-free, 1 cup	625
Sweet potato, baked, with skin, medium	542
100% orange juice, 8 ounces	496
Broccoli, chopped, cooked, 1 cup	457
Low-fat (1%) chocolate milk, 8 ounces	425
Banana, 1 medium	422
Cantaloupe, cubed, 1 cup	417
Milk, fat-free, 8 ounces	382
Navy beans, canned, drained, ½ cup	377
Lentils, cooked, ½ cup	365
Pork tenderloin, cooked, 3 ounces	358

Food	Potassium (mg)
Salmon, farmed, Atlantic, cooked, 3 ounces	326
California raisins, ¼ cup	299
Pistachios, shelled, 1 ounce	285
Mango, chopped, 1 cup	277
Cod, Atlantic, cooked, 3 ounces	207
Almonds, 1 ounce	200

Source: USDA

Get Your Fill of Fiber

What's up with fiber? Your body's incapable of digesting it, yet fiber is an important part of the diet. Fiber, found naturally in plant foods, helps to protect against cardiovascular disease, type 2 diabetes, and constipation. Fiber helps you feel fuller for longer, so it encourages weight control.

Daily fiber requirements are tied to calorie needs. Aim for 14 grams of fiber for every 1,000 calories you need to maintain your weight or for weight loss. For example, include 28 grams of fiber a day on a 2,000-calorie eating plan. Children who need about 1,400 calories a day require about 20 grams of fiber daily. Don't go overboard on high-fiber foods for children. The fact that fiber is filling is actually one of its failings when it comes to young kids. Excess fiber in a child's diet may decrease his appetite for foods that provide the calories he needs to grow and develop properly.

Fiber-Filled Foods

Fiber is found in fruits, vegetables, beans, peas, nuts, and grains. To easily reach your daily fiber quota, include foods with fiber at every meal and snack. Use the Nutrition Facts Panel label to look for grams of fiber per serving.

Food	Fiber (grams)
Raspberries, 1 cup	8
Beans (navy, pinto, black, kidney, white, great northern, lima), cooked, ½ cup	6-9
Split peas, lentils, chickpeas, cowpeas, cooked, ½ cup	6-8
Pear, medium	6
Soybeans, cooked, ½ cup	5
Breakfast cereal, ready-to-eat, 1 cup	5-10

Food	Fiber (grams)
Whole-wheat English muffin, 2 ounces	4
Apple, with skin, 1 medium	4
Sweet potato, baked, medium	4
Figs, dried, ¼ cup	4
Potato, baked, with skin, medium	4
Almonds, 1 ounce	4
Strawberries, sliced, 1 cup	3
Banana, 1 medium	3
Pistachios, shelled, 1 ounce	3
California raisins, ¼ cup	3
Mango, sliced, 1 cup	3
Whole-wheat bread, 1 slice	2

Source: USDA

Nutrients of Special Concern

Women in their childbearing years and people over the age of 50 should pay special attention to certain nutrients, according to the Dietary Guidelines. Women need to get the iron and folate/folic acid that they require every day, and older people need a certain type of vitamin B12.

Your body may not adequately absorb vitamin B12 after age 50, even if you get the suggested daily amount that occurs naturally in food. Here's why: Older people don't produce as much stomach acid, which is necessary to free the natural form of vitamin B12 from food and make it available to the body for absorption.

The 2010 Dietary Guidelines recommend that adults over 50 years of age get most of the suggested daily vitamin B12, which is 2.4 micrograms (mcg), from fortified foods or dietary supplements containing vitamin B12. The form of vitamin B12 in fortified foods and dietary supplements does not require stomach acid to assist in absorption.

You should still include foods rich in vitamin B because they offer other nutrients, too. Vitamin B12 is present naturally in animal products, including meat, poultry, seafood, milk, and eggs. If you skip animal foods, or skimp on them, fortified foods and dietary supplements are helpful for fulfilling the recommended daily amounts of vitamin B12.

Here are some of the best sources of vitamin B12.

Food	Vitamin B12 (micrograms)
Breakfast cereals, fortified with 100% of the Daily Value for vitamin B12, 1 serving	6
Trout, rainbow, wild, cooked, 3 ounces	5.4
Salmon, sockeye, cooked, 3 ounces	4.2
Beef, top sirloin, cooked, 3 ounces	2.4
Yogurt, plain, low-fat, 1 cup	1.4
Egglands Best egg, 1 large	1.3
Tuna, white, canned, 3 ounces	1
Milk, low-fat (1%), 8 ounces	1
Egg, large, 1 whole	.6
Chicken breast, meat only, cooked, 3½ ounces	.34

Source: USDA

Get More for Your Calories, and Your Food Dollar

Chances are, you lack the time or the motivation (or both!) to tally grams of fiber and count up micrograms of vitamin B12 to help yourself and your family to eat better. No worries! After all, you eat food, not nutrients.

Including more nutrient-rich foods, such as fruit, vegetables, whole grains, fat-free and low-fat dairy, and lean protein sources helps you fill in dietary gaps for the four major missing nutrients, and many more.

Nutrient-rich foods provide the biggest nutritional bang for your caloric buck, because they supply the most nutrients for the least calories, relatively speaking. Many nutrient-rich foods are budget-friendly, too. For example, eight ounces of fat-free milk supplies about one-third of an adult's calcium needs for the day for about twenty-five cents and 100 calories a serving. One foritifed egg, such as Eggland's Best, costs about the same as milk, but provides twice as much vitamin A and vitamin D and ten times as much vitamin E as a regular egg. And a half-cup serving of beans, which will set you back less than 50 cents, serves up protein, fiber, vitamins, and minerals for a small amount of money.

When you choose nutrient-rich foods more often, you can eat less food to get the good nutrition you need. Eating less food means saving more money.

MyPlate's Messages

MyPlate is clear on what types of nutrient-rich foods to choose. Here's more on why MyPlate's recommendations are worthy of your attention.

Dairy Foods: Choose fat-free and low-fat (1%) milk.

You may think milk is just for kids. It's not. Children and adults need dairy foods their entire lives to bolster bone health, and for other reasons. Milk and other vitamin-D fortified dairy foods contribute three out the four nutrients missing from the typical American eating plan: calcium, vitamin D, and potassium. Some evidence suggests that milk products are linked to a lower risk of cardiovascular disease and type 2 diabetes, and that they help to reduce blood pressure in adults.

The recommendations made by MyPlate for milk and milk products, which, technically speaking, include milk, yogurt, fortified soy beverages, and cheese, refer to fat-free and low-fat (1%) products. (Foods made from milk that have little or no calcium, such as cream cheese, cream, and butter, are not part of the dairy group.) Higher-fat dairy foods are not necessarily off-limits, but you should make allowances in your diet for the extra fat and calories they contain. The same goes for flavored milk; it serves up some added sugar, but that doesn't mean you must eliminate it. Instead, account for the extra 56 calories and 14 grams of sugar in an eight-ounce glass.

Nearly half of the milk and milk product intake in the American diet comes from cheese. Cheese is good for you. The problem is, cheese can be high in total and saturated fat, and sodium. Cheese made with less sodium or fat is a good choice because it offers the same amount of protein and calcium. You won't find vitamin D in most cheese, however. The same goes for yogurt, although some brands may contain vitamin D. Look on the Nutrient Facts panel, and opt for yogurt that provides at least 20% of the Daily Value for vitamin D, which amounts to 120 International Units of vitamin D, a bit more than a glass of milk.

Soy beverages are an acceptable alternative to cow's milk as long as they contain as much calcium, and vitamins A and D, as milk. If you're lactose intolerant, rely on lactose-free milk and dairy products, such as Lactaid brand, so that you can enjoy milk and get all the benefits it offers without the lactose.

 ## Milk On the Menu

MyPlate milk recommendations are based on age. Children ages 12 months to two years need full-fat milk for the calories, fat, and cholesterol it provides. Most children over the age of two can drink low-fat (1%) milk and fat-free milk. Here's what you and your kids need every day:

- Children ages 2 to 3 years: 16 ounces (2 cups)
- Children ages four to eight years: 20 ounces (2½ cups)
- Everyone ages nine and above: 24 ounces (3 cups)

It's not necessary to drink milk or a fortified soy beverage straight up. There are plenty of ways to work a serving of milk (8 ounces) into the menu:

- Prepare oatmeal and other cooked cereals with fat-free or low-fat milk (1%) in the microwave.
- Make pudding mix with fat-free or low-fat (1%) milk.
- Sip a smoothie made with 8 ounces of milk or low-fat yogurt and fruit.
- Enjoy 12 ounces of a latte or cappuccino to get the benefits of 8 ounces of milk. Make it with fat-free milk and decaf coffee, if desired.
- Prepare reduced-sodium condensed soups with milk instead of water.
- Enjoy yogurt and fruit for a snack.
- Make hot chocolate (using a mix) with milk instead of water.
- Add a slice of low-fat or reduced-fat cheese to your sandwich.
- Cook with low-fat cottage cheese or enjoy it as a dip with vegetables.

Fruits and Vegetables: Make half your plate fruits and vegetables.
Do you eat enough fruits and vegetables? Do your kids? Probably
not. The American diet is short on produce, and MyPlate says it's
time we changed that.

Fruits and vegetables supply potassium and fiber, two of the
four major missing nutrients in most people's diets. Plus, produce
is cholesterol-free and most is naturally low in fat, sodium, and
calories. Here are the other benefits these plant foods provide:

- Fruits and vegetables are rich in the B vitamin folate, magne-
  sium, vitamins C and K, and beta-carotene, a pigment that provides color and acts to protect cells in your body against damage.
- Eating at least 2½ cups of fruits and vegetables daily is linked
  to a lower risk of heart attack and stroke, and some produce may
  be protective against certain types of cancer in adults.
- When prepared and eaten without added fats or sugars, fruits
  and veggies are relatively low in calories for the nutrients they
  provide, and they can help you, and your children, achieve and
  maintain a healthy weight.
- Produce provides fiber. Diets rich in foods containing fiber may
  reduce the risk of heart disease, obesity, and type 2 diabetes.
  Fiber also helps promote proper bowel function.
- Fruits and veggies supply potassium, which, as part of a healthy
  diet, may lower blood pressure, and may also reduce the risk of
  developing kidney stones and protect bones.

Eat More, and Vary Your Fruits and Vegetables
The amount of produce you should eat every day depends on how
many total calories you eat. Active adults and teens need about five
servings of fruits and vegetables, and younger children should eat
between two and three servings a day.

In general, 1 cup of fruit, ½ cup of dried fruit, or 100% fruit
juice counts as a serving of fruit. Fruits may be fresh, canned,
frozen, or dried, and may be whole, cut-up, or pureed.

When it comes to vegetables, 1 cup of raw or cooked vegetables
or vegetable juice, or two cups of raw leafy greens is considered a
serving. Vegetables may be raw or cooked; fresh, frozen, canned,
dried, or dehydrated; and may be whole, cut-up, or mashed.

MyPlate's main message about produce is to fill half your plate
with fruits and vegetables. That's the first step to healthier eating.

Next is to focus on variety:

Experts say you should vary the types of produce you eat as much as possible, for the simple reason that while fruits and vegetables have many common nutrients, they differ nutritionally in important ways. For example, beans and peas are rich in protein, which most vegetables lack. In addition, beans and peas supply iron and zinc in amounts similar to seafood, meat, and poultry. On the other hand, beans and peas aren't particularly high in vitamin C, but citrus fruits, kiwi,

Vary the types of produce you eat as much as possible, for the simple reason that while fruits and vegetables have many common nutrients, they differ nutritionally in important ways.

◻ Vegetables Are Not Created Equal

Are some vegetables better than others? Strictly speaking, yes. Darker greens, such as Romaine lettuce and spinach have more nutrients than iceberg lettuce, for example. However, every vegetable has something to offer, so if you only like a few vegetables, make sure to include them every day in amounts that contribute to meeting your daily produce needs.

and tomatoes are rich in this important nutrient. Sweet potatoes and carrots are packed with beta-carotene, which provides their orange hue, is a potent antioxidant that protects cells against damage, and serves as the raw material for making vitamin A.

Vegetables are divided up into five groups: starchy, dark green, red and orange, beans and peas, and other vegetables. With the exception of "other vegetables," the headings aptly describe the members in each category. To learn more about each of these groups, visit ChooseMyPlate.gov/food-groups/vegetables.html

◻ In the Red

Tomato products are among the richest vegetables in potassium, and tomatoes are also a favorite among Americans. Tomato products, including canned chopped tomatoes, tomato sauce, and tomato paste, are available year-round. They're versatile and convenient to use in a number of dishes including chili, pasta dishes, sauces, soups, stews, and pizza. Choose tomato products and juices labeled "no salt added," "reduced sodium," and "low sodium."

Gobble the Garden:
How to Eat More Fruits and Vegetables

There are a lot of reasons why we don't get the recommended fruits and vegetables every day, including lack of time and lack of interest in eating them. Here are some solutions, including time-saving tips and ways to make produce more interesting and readily available to you and your family.

- Buy seasonal fruits and vegetables. They're less expensive and are likely to taste better.

- Keep frozen fruits and vegetables on hand. You can't eat produce if it's not available.

- Stock up on dried fruit, such as California raisins, cranberries, and apricots to add to snacks, main dishes, and desserts. Keep some in your bag for a quick snack.

- Capitalize on convenience and buy pre-cut fruits and vegetables. Or, save money by cutting them at home.

- Top breakfast cereal with berries, bananas, or dried fruit.

- Add berries to pancakes, and use applesauce to top waffles, pancakes, and crepes instead of syrup.

- Always opt for 100% fruit juice, such as orange juice, instead of sugary juice beverages.

- Add crushed pineapple to coleslaw and toss chopped grapes with chicken and tuna salad.

- Offer kids half of a peanut butter or sunflower seed butter sandwich with sliced banana or apple on whole-wheat bread.

- Spread almond butter on sliced apples or pears for a snack.

- Puree fruit, such as fresh mango or canned apricots and combine with fat-free or low-fat plain yogurt.

- Make your own trail mix with chopped almonds, walnuts, pistachios or sunflower seeds, whole-grain cereal, and dried fruit.

- Make fruit kabobs with pineapple chunks, bananas, grapes, and berries.

- Always order fruit when dining out at fast food chains or any restaurant.

- Sip 100% vegetable juice with a meal or as a snack.

- Set a good example for your children by including a salad and fruit with dinner every night to help make half your plate fruits and vegetables.

- Plan meals around vegetables, such as a vegetable and beef or chicken stir-fry or chili. Double the amount of vegetables and reduce meat by half in your favorite recipe.

More ideas next page...

Continued from previous page...

- Keep a bowl full of fruit on the counter. Place a container of cut-up vegetables in a see-through container in the refrigerator with low-fat dips, such as Ranch dressing and hummus, on hand for dipping.
- Get kids involved with fruit and vegetable choices. Allow them to pick a vegetable to have at home while shopping.
- Make veggie pizzas at home using chopped red bell pepper, mushrooms, onions, and artichokes. When ordering pizza, ask for extra vegetables.
- Stock up on frozen vegetables so that you can prepare what you need without waste.
- Add a 14-ounce can of cooked pumpkin or other pureed cooked vegetables, such as sweet potato, to stews, soups, and gravies. Pureed vegetables add flavor, nutrients, and texture.
- Add chopped vegetables to prepared pasta sauce or to your favorite lasagna recipe.
- Pack fruits and vegetables with every meal and snack you eat away from home.
- Roast vegetables, such as chopped broccoli and cauliflower, and thickly-sliced carrots. Toss with olive oil and the herbs of your choice and roast at 400°F for about 15 to 20 minutes.
- When roasting meat, throw one or two sweet potatoes in the oven to have later for snacks or with a meal.
- Grill vegetables, such as asparagus and eggplant. Brush each piece with olive oil before setting directly on the grill.
- Try grilled fruit.
- Buy fruits canned in water or 100% juice so that you always have a supply on hand. Individual containers of fruits like peaches or applesauce are easy and convenient.
- Prepare fruit-based desserts, such as fruit crisp, baked apples or pears, or fruit salad.
- Make frozen juice bars with 100% fruit. They are less expensive than store-bought and more fun for the kids.
- Start the day with 8 ounces of 100% orange juice. Kids under six can have 6 ounces.
- Pack a juice box (100% juice) in children's lunches instead of soda or other sugar-sweetened beverages.
- Forgo chewy fruit snacks and offer kids whole fruit instead. There is often little fruit in "fruit-flavored" treats.
- Include salsa with meals or have as a snack. Make your own fruit or vegetable salsa.

Beans and Peas: Doubly good, and more

Beans and peas—including kidney beans, pinto beans, black beans, garbanzo beans (chickpeas), lima beans, black-eyed peas, split peas, and lentils—are the vegetables with the most protein and fiber. They're also packed with so many other nutrients that they are considered both a vegetable and a protein food.

You may not have grown up eating a lot of beans, or maybe they were relegated to side dishes. Kids love beans, so offer them a variety. Here's how to include more beans in your MyPlate plan for better eating.

- Replace meat with beans for meatless chili or pasta dishes.
- Mix black beans (and frozen, thawed corn) to store-bought salsa to create a tasty black bean salsa.
- Add a can of drained beans to pasta sauce and serve over whole-wheat pasta.
- Choose bean-based soups and stews, such as lentil and vegetarian chili, instead of chicken noodle.
- Keep canned beans on hand to add to salads, soups, and pasta dishes or to eat for snacks.
- Snack on salsa, hummus, or black bean dip and low-fat crackers or baked snack chips instead of potato chips and other snack chips.

Whole Grains: Make at least half your grains whole.

Any food made from wheat, rice, oats, cornmeal, barley, or another cereal grain is a grain product. Experts divide grains into whole grains and refined grains. Whole grains, such as oatmeal and brown rice, contain the entire grain kernel. Refined grains, including white bread and white rice, have been milled, which removes the bran and germ.

The recommended number of grain servings you should have each day depends on your calorie needs. Active adults and teens need about seven servings of grains daily, while younger children require about four to five servings. In general, 1 slice of bread, 1 cup of ready-to-eat cereal, or ½ cup of cooked rice, cooked pasta, or cooked cereal can be considered as a 1 ounce equivalent from the Grains Group, also known as a serving. No matter how many servings of grains are in your healthy diet, you should make at least half of them whole grains.

Do you eat enough whole grains? If you do, you're part of a very small group. Only 15% of Americans include the recommended three servings or more of whole grains every day. That's a shame, because whole grains are full of health benefits, the least of which is that they reduce the risk of cardiovascular disease and are linked a lower risk of type 2 diabetes. Whole grains help with weight control, and they are naturally richer in dietary fiber, iron, and B vitamins.

How to include more whole grains
- *Substitute 100% whole-grain breads, cereals, rice, pasta, and crackers at meals and snacks for refined choices.*
- *Add whole grains, such as whole-grain barley or cracked wheat to mixed dishes such as soups, stews, and casseroles.*
- *Try whole-wheat pasta, quinoa, or farro for a change of pace.*
- *Snack on popcorn instead of pretzels or chips. Popcorn is a whole grain.*
- *Substitute whole-wheat flour for up to half of the white flour in your favorite quick bread recipes such as pancakes, waffles, and muffins.*
- *Snack on whole-grain cereal mixed with dried fruit and nuts, or have a small bowl of whole-grain ready-to-eat cereal or oatmeal for a snack.*

Hunting for Whole Grains
You can't tell a whole grain by its color or its fiber content, although many whole grains are darker and contain more fiber than refined. Choose foods with one of the following terms listed first in the ingredient list:

- Whole wheat
- Brown rice
- Bulgur
- Oatmeal
- Rolled oats
- Whole-grain corn
- Whole-grain triticale
- Wild rice
- Buckwheat
- Millet
- Quinoa
- Whole-grain barley
- Whole-grain sorghum
- Whole oats

Foods labeled with the words "multi-grain," "stone-ground," "100% wheat," "cracked wheat," "seven-grain," or "bran" are typically not whole-grain products.

Eat More of This

MyPlate's intent is positive. It's all about including nutrient-rich foods, not about what to leave off your plate, or out of your cup. Focusing on what you can eat decreases feelings of deprivation and allows you to focus on what you can do to make your diet, and your family's, better.

Of course, there are some foods you should limit. That's the focus of the next chapter. Not to worry. Healthy eating involves enjoyments, so there's always room for fun!

CHAPTER 5

What Not to Eat

YOU'RE TIRED OF ADVICE about what not to eat, and that's understandable. Being told to cut back on your favorite high-calorie foods is a downer, and it pays to be positive about what to include in your diet.

But you knew some discussion of what to avoid was coming, right?

So here's a promise, upfront: This chapter, which does contain information about foods to curb, will be brief, entertaining, and useful. And you may be pleasantly surprised to find that there is no need to exclude all your favorite foods in the name of better health. Promise.

Solid Fats and Added Sugars: The Usual Suspects

Americans consume a whopping 35% of their energy—about 800 calories every day- from solid fats and added sugar (SoFAS) in foods and beverages. That's more than double what the 2010 Dietary Guidelines recommend for most children and adults.

Foods with added sugars or solid fats, such as butter, shortening, and lard, or both, are no more likely to contribute to overweight and obesity than other foods, as long as you stick to your calorie allowance, that is. So why are nutrition experts concerned about them? Because most people eat more calories than they need, and many of those calories come from food with added sugars, added solid fats, or both.

In addition to possibly adding excess calories, as the amount of solid fats and/or added sugars rises

> ### ⬛ Solid Fat Hit Parade
>
> The major sources of solid fats in the typical American diet include cookies, cakes, pastry, pizza, full-fat cheese, sausage, franks, bacon, ribs, and fried white potatoes.

in your diet, it's difficult to include foods with the vitamins, minerals, and fiber you need without busting your daily calorie allowance. There's simply no room left for healthier foods.

While fatty and/or sugary fare often crowds out more nutritious choices, some foods with solid fats are highly nutritious and shouldn't be demonized for their fat content.

While fatty and/or sugary fare often crowds out more nutritious choices, some foods with solid fats are highly nutritious and shouldn't be demonized for their fat content.

The fat in fluid milk is considered a solid fat by Dietary Guideline standards because milk fat is solid at room temperature. (Milk fat is suspended in fluid milk through the process of homogenization.) Plain milk, no matter what fat level, is packed with protein, B vitamins, phosphorus, calcium, and vitamins A and D. Flavored fat-free and low-fat (1%) milk, which contains added sugar, is an example of a sweet, yet highly nutritious food. One glass of fat-free chocolate milk supplies 56 more calories than plain because of some added sugar, but contributes exactly the same levels of protein, vitamins, and minerals, especially the calcium and vitamin D that are missing from children's diets.

Certain cuts of beef, such as 85% lean ground beef, supply more solid fat, but provide an excellent source of protein, iron, and zinc. Cheese is another example of a protein- and calcium-rich food with substantial solid fat.

Portions matter. Enjoying smaller servings of any food helps you better control your calorie intake and reduce the solid fats and added sugars you consume. Lower-fat and lower-sugar versions of favorite foods help you decrease your intake of solid fats or added sugars, too.

We may be way off the mark when it comes to our solid fats and sugar intake, but the fact that the 2010 Dietary Guidelines, and MyPlate, provide for any solid fats and added sugars in a balanced diet suggests that while a lot of solid fat and added sugar is hazardous to your health, a little won't hurt you. For example, on a 2,000-calorie diet, you're allowed to include 258 calories worth of SoFAS a day, the amount found in about a half cup of premium ice cream. Younger children, who tend to eat less, can have about 120 calories worth of solid fat and added sugar on a 1,400-calorie eating plan, which amounts to a little less than an ounce of snack chips or three sandwich cookies.

Spotlight on Solid Fats

Fats that are solid at room temperature occur naturally in food (such as the marbling in beef and the fat in cheese) and are also used as ingredients in packaged foods. The fats in meat, poultry, and eggs are considered solid fats, while the fats in seafood, nuts, and seeds are considered oils. At nine calories per gram, solid fat provides twice the calories of carbohydrate and protein, and, in most cases, supplies unhealthy saturated fat and trans fatty acids, too.

Solid fats are responsible for an average of 20% of our total calorie intake, but provide nothing much in the way of nutrition. Reducing solid fat intake without adding calories from other food puts a dent in your energy consumption and slashes saturated and trans fatty acid intake, which is beneficial to your health, and your child's.

Solid fats include:

- Butter
- Chicken fat
- Stick margarine
- Coconut oil
- Beef fat (tallow, suet)
- Pork fat (lard)
- Shortening
- Palm oil

Give Added Sugars The Slip

Every gram of extra sugar in foods adds four calories. It pays to read the Nutrition Facts panel, and check the ingredients list, as added sugar goes by many names. Don't assume that "naturally-sweetened" means low in sugar. Look for the many aliases for sugar on food labels:

- anhydrous dextrose
- brown sugar
- cane juice
- confectioner's powdered sugar
- corn syrup
- corn syrup solids
- crystal dextrose
- dextrin
- evaporated corn sweetener
- fructose
- fruit juice concentrate
- fruit nectar
- glucose
- high-fructose corn syrup
- honey
- invert sugar
- lactose*
- liquid fructose
- malt syrup
- maltose

List continued to the next page...

Lactose is the naturally occurring sugar in dairy foods. It is not added sugar, but because it is a simple sugar, it is listed with Sugars on the Nutrient Facts panel.

...continued from previous page

- maple syrup
- molasses
- nectars (peach nectar, pear nectar, etc.)
- pancake syrup
- raw sugar
- sucrose
- sugar
- sugar cane juice
- white granulated sugar

The Low-down On Low-calorie Sweeteners

Sugar substitutes, such as sucralose, saccharin, and aspartame, are useful for curbing calories and controlling blood glucose (sugar) levels. You may also notice sweeteners with names like xylitol, mannitol, and sorbitol on food labels. These are sugar alcohols, but they don't contain ethanol like alcoholic beverages. Sugar alcohols provide up to half the calories of sugar, so they are not calorie-free.

Should you feed yourself and your kids foods sweetened with low-calorie sugar substitutes? That depends. Calorie-free sugar substitutes are a boon to people with diabetes, who need to closely monitor their carbohydrate intake. There is some controversy surrounding the safety of low-calorie sweeteners, so you many not want your children to consume them on a regular basis, especially if they don't need to. Plus, sugar alcohols can cause diarrhea, gas, and intestinal discomfort.

Also, keep in mind that foods made with sugar substitutes are not always calorie-free, nor are they rich in the essential nutrients that adults and kids need. Some sugar is permissible, and it may be wiser to choose foods that are sweetened with natural, calorie-free alternatives, such as monk fruit concentrate. Monk fruit is a traditional food found in Asia, and it's being used, in a concentrated form, to replace some of the sugar in popular foods. Look for drinks, dairy products, breakfast cereals, bars, baked goods, and candy sweetened with monk fruit for options with less sugar and fewer calories.

Grains: We're Too Refined

We love our grains. Grain-based desserts, such as cookies, cake, and yeast breads, including white, mixed-grain, and whole-wheat bread, bagels, and rolls, top the list of calorie contributors in the diets of Americans ages two and older.

We eat a lot of grains, but they're not the right type. In all like-lihood, the bulk of your grain intake is refined. MyPlate recommends that half of your daily grain servings—a minimum of three servings, such as one slice of bread or ½ cup cooked grain—come from whole grains.

Here's why you should give refined grains the shaft, at least half the time. Refined grains are milled, resulting in a finer texture and a longer shelf life. Those are desirable traits, for consumers and for food manufacturers. But there's a downside to refining: the loss of vitamins, minerals, and dietary fiber. To make matters worse, many of the refined grains we eat, including cookies, cake, and crackers, are also rich in solid fats and/or added sugars, adding to the calorie count.

Refined grains include:
- White flour
- White bread, crackers, and rolls
- White rice
- Couscous
- Pasta
- Donuts and other pastry
- Cookies
- Pretzels
- Cake
- Degermed cornmeal
- Cornbread
- Flour and corn tortillas
- Certain ready-to-eat cereals (check the ingredient list for whole grains)

Despite their downside, refined grains have admirable qualities. All grains, including the refined kind, are rich in carbohydrate, the body's preferred energy source. Many refined grains, such as white rice and pasta, are naturally low in fat, and several, such as breakfast cereals, bread, rice, and pasta, supply added iron and added B vitamins, including folic acid, which is helpful in preventing certain birth defects early in pregnancy. Enriched grains are a major source of *non-heme* iron for Americans, particularly children, and they are useful in heading off iron deficiency and iron deficiency anemia.

Alcohol

About half of American adults are regular drinkers, which may be beneficial—or not. Alcoholic beverages can be calorie budget busters, especially when your daily calorie allowance is in the lower range. An occasional drink won't make a difference in your waist-line, but calories from alcoholic beverages must be accounted for in your calorie budget if you drink on a regular basis. See page 104 for more on how much alcohol is enough and why alcohol may be good for you and when it's a health hazard.

Sodium: Get the salt out?

Sodium gets a bad rap as being a health buster. But that overly simplistic take on sodium does not do it justice. You need sodium to keep your body running properly. Sodium promotes fluid balance in the body, and fosters proper cell function.

Most everyone ages two and older consumes about twice the sodium suggested in the 2010 Dietary Guidelines— however, the bulk of the sodium we eat doesn't come from the salt shaker.

Here's the problem: Our sodium intake is way over the top, and salt, a major source of sodium, is the primary culprit. Most everyone ages two and older consumes about twice the sodium suggested in the 2010 Dietary Guidelines. The bulk of the sodium we eat doesn't come from the salt shaker, however. Most of the salt consumed is from packaged foods and restaurant fare.

The Dietary Guidelines recommends limiting our sodium intake to less than 2,300 milligrams (mg) a day, and MyPlate suggests including foods lower in sodium as much as possible. If you fall into one of the following groups, which includes about half of the U.S. population, the suggested limit is 1,500 mg of sodium daily:

- Over the age of 51
- African American, any age
- Have high blood pressure (hypertension), diabetes, or chronic kidney disease

Why should children be mindful of sodium? As sodium intake increases in adults and children, so does blood pressure. High blood pressure is linked to increased risk of heart disease, stroke, and kidney failure. Blood pressure naturally rises with age, and African Americans are more prone to elevated blood pressure. That's why the Dietary Guidelines recommends lower amounts of sodium for these groups. If you have high blood pressure, diabetes, or chronic kidney failure, reducing sodium intake to the suggested lower levels will help to manage these conditions.

Sodium doesn't supply calories, so it can't contribute to excess weight and obesity. However, the more food you consume, the higher your sodium intake. That makes sense when you consider that sodium is present in nearly everything you eat. Since most adults and many children are overweight, they naturally consume more sodium because they overeat. Eating less, and eating fewer salty foods, can significantly slash sodium intake.

Seeking Sodium

The Nutrition Facts Panel on food labels is an excellent source of sodium information. It provides the number of milligrams of sodium per serving in foods and beverages. Seeking out sodium amounts is trickier when it comes to restaurant foods and salty seasonings. Here's a list of sodium-rich foods that may or may not carry labels.

Food	Sodium (mg)
Salt, 1 teaspoon	2,325
Cold cut sandwich, 6-inch roll, fast food	1,651
Taco, large, fast food	1,233
Biscuit, egg, sausage sandwich, fast food	1,210
Ham, 3 ounces	1,128
Soy sauce, 1 tablespoon	902
Cheeseburger, with condiments, fast food	843
Pasta sauce, marinara, ½ cup	512

Sources: USDA

Salt and Sensibility: What's Good About Salt

When you use salt at home, make sure it's the iodized kind. The mineral iodine is a major part of thyroid hormones that regulate key bodily functions, including your metabolic rate. During pregnancy, iodine is crucial for proper brain and nervous system development. Goiter, the enlargement of the thyroid gland, is the result of inadequate iodine intake.

Foods such as seafood, and plants grown in soil that contains iodine, are sources of this mighty mineral. So is the meat from animals that eat plants grown in iodine-containing soil. The level of iodine in soil varies, and few people eat the likes of cod, sea bass, haddock, and perch on a regular basis, so you may come up short for iodine.

Iodized salt fills the void. According to the Salt Institute, household use of iodized salt has essentially eliminated iodine deficiency in North America. The Salt Institute estimates that nearly

70% of the table salt sold in the U.S. is iodized. That's the good news about iodine.

The bad news is that it's uncertain if processed foods contain iodized salt. Using plain salt that isn't iodized can lead to an iodine deficiency. That's cause for concern, as Americans don't cook at home as often as they once did and rely more heavily on packaged and prepared foods. The irony is that packaged and processed fare is so salty, yet may not provide us with the iodine we need. The solution: Cook more at home, and use a smattering of iodized salt.

Subtract Some Sodium

When you gradually reduce the sodium in your foods, you may lose your preference for saltiness. You don't need to count every milligram of sodium to subtract some sodium from your eating pattern. You can make a substantial dent in salt intake by using these tips on a daily basis.

- Focus on eating more fresh and lightly-processed foods.
- MyPlate recommends comparing the sodium levels of foods such as soup, bread, and frozen meals. Select products labeled "low sodium," "reduced sodium," or "no salt added."

- When dining out, ask that no salt, or other salty ingredients, such as soy sauce and MSG (monosodium glutamate) be added to your foods, and choose lower sodium options, such as a baked potato instead of French fries and a fresh salad instead of soup. Peruse restaurant web sites and menu information for sodium content before you arrive at a restaurant.
- Substitute lemon juice, spices, and spice blends for some or all of the salt when cooking at home.

Spice It Up

Spices are sodium-free and they make food more interesting by adding flavor as well as antioxidants, plant compounds that protect cells from damage.

- **Ground cinnamon:** Add 1¼ teaspoons to prepared 1-minute oatmeal; to 1 cup Greek yogurt mixed with 2 teaspoons molasses or honey; or to French toast batter. Sprinkle ½ teaspoon cinnamon over ground coffee before brewing, or top a fat-free latte or hot cocoa with ground cinnamon.
- **Chili peppers:** Add chopped peppers to chili, burgers, soups, stews, salsa, and egg dishes.
- **Turmeric:** Sprinkle on egg salad. Mix ½ teaspoon with 1 cup plain Greek yogurt and use as a dip or sandwich spread. Add to chicken or seafood casseroles and to water when cooking rice.
- **Garlic:** Add fresh chopped or minced garlic to pasta dishes, stir-fry dishes, pizza, fresh tomato sauce, and meat and poultry recipes.
- **Oregano:** Add ⅛ teaspoon dried to scrambled eggs, salad dressings, or store-bought and homemade marinara sauce. Sprinkle some dried or fresh oregano on top of pizza or stir into black bean soup.
- **Basil:** Make a sandwich with low-fat mozzarella cheese, sliced tomatoes, and fresh basil leaves; add fresh basil leaves to green salads.
- **Thyme:** Sprinkle dried thyme onto cooked vegetables in place of butter or margarine. Add ⅛ teaspoon dried thyme to two scrambled eggs and to salad dressings, or use it in a rub when cooking salmon. Add fresh or dried thyme to chicken salad and chicken soup.
- **Rosemary:** Add dried crushed rosemary to mashed potatoes and vegetable omelets.
- **Parsley:** Add chopped flat leaf parsley to meatballs and meat loaf, and to bulgur salad.

More spices next page...

...Continued from previous page

- **Ginger:** Grate fresh ginger into quick bread batters and vinaigrette, add chopped ginger to stir-fries, and sprinkle ground ginger on cooked carrots.
- **Cloves:** Sprinkle ground cloves on applesauce, add to quick bread batters, and add a pinch to hot tea.

That's a Wrap

That wasn't so bad, was it? Following MyPlate eating recommendations doesn't rule out favorite foods such as ice cream, cookies, chips, beer, or snack chips. As you can see, you can have the foods you love, within reason, of course. Next up: all about fat, what types to include, and how much.

CHAPTER 6

The Facts About Fat and Cholesterol

FAT IS NOT A FOUR-LETTER WORD, but it might as well be. We have a love/hate relationship with fat: we love the way it makes food taste, but we hate what it can do to our bodies, including its contributions to expanding waistlines and clogged arteries.

While fat may be guilty on both counts, it's not entirely fair to convict all fats since the amount and types of fat you eat is what influences your health. Even if you're not overweight, consuming too much of the wrong types of fat may put you at risk for heart disease, one of the most common chronic conditions in the United States.

Fats (also known as lipids) are complex and are deserving of special attention. In this chapter, you'll learn how much fat to eat and discover the details about cholesterol and different types of fat.

> ### ☐ It's the Calories, Silly!
>
> Dietary fat doesn't translate into excess body fat any more than the carbohydrate or protein in your diet. Total calorie intake is what matters most when it comes to weight control.

Why Fat Does a Body Good

Fat in the diet provides energy and the raw materials for compounds that promote wellbeing. Here are some of the ways fat works in the body.

- *Contributes a concentrated source of calories:* Fat supplies nine calories per gram, more than double that of carbohydrate or protein. Babies, infants, and toddlers, whose energy needs are high relative to their weight, require such a concentrated calorie source to grow and develop properly. As much as we curse its caloric content, it would be difficult for most adults to meet their daily calorie quotas without fat in their eating plans, too.

- *Provides essential fatty acids (EFA):* Good health would be impossible without dietary fat. Fat in food provides the EFAs linoleic acid and alpha-linolenic acid. EFA are compounds that your body cannot make on its own, and that are essential to life.
- *Ferries fat-soluble vitamins:* You need dietary fat to bolster the absorption and transportation of fat-soluble substances including vitamins A, D, E, and K, and carotenoids, which provide the raw materials to make vitamin A in the body, and act as antioxidants.
- *Promotes brain development and vision:* Fat, most notably, docosahexaenoic acid (DHA), makes up part of the cells in the brain and the retina, the portion of the eye that registers images and relays the information to the brain for processing. DHA is especially important during pregnancy and infancy to provide your child with what he needs for peak brain development and vision.

You're a Fat Head

About 60% of your brain is fat. Fat is a component of cell membranes, the outer layer of cells, and it's part of myelin, the protective sheath that surrounds nerve cells in the brain and throughout the body. Docosahexaenoic acid (DHA), a kind of fat found in seafood and fortified foods, is the dominant type found in the brain.

Dietary Fat: The Basic Facts

Now you know: you need fat. But what's the best type, and how much should you have?

Fat contains a combination of saturated, trans, monounsaturated, and polyunsaturated fatty acids. All foods have a mixture of fats, but one type always prevails and tends to be associated with that food. For example, butter is associated with foods rich in saturated fat, while olive oil is classified as a food with unsaturated fat.

Here are the basic facts about the different fat types:

Saturated fat: Your body makes all the saturated fat it needs to get by, which is why you don't need any from food. That's not to say you can't have some saturated fat every day. The 2010 Dietary Guidelines suggest limiting saturated fat intake to 10% or less of your total calories, about 22 grams or less in a 2,000-calorie diet.

Eating more than the recommended amount of saturated fat may result in higher total and LDL ("bad" cholesterol) in your bloodstream and may lead to clogged arteries that could block the flow of oxygen-rich blood to your heart and brain. Eating 7% or less of your calories as saturated fat (about 16 grams or less on a 2,000-calorie diet) helps to further reduce the risk of cardiovascular disease.

Saturated fat is the most prevalent kind of fat in higher-calorie cuts of meat, full-fat milk and cheese, butter, coconut oil and butter, and palm oil and palm kernel oil. However, it's unnecessary to completely avoid foods with saturated fats in the name of heart health.

Foods such as meat, milk, and cheese offer protein, vitamins, and minerals that you and your family need. To keep saturated fat within the suggested guidelines, eat smaller portions of foods rich in saturated fat, such as full-fat cheese, the number one source of saturated fat in the American diet. You should also substitute lower-fat options, such as fat-free and low-fat (1%) milk, reduced fat cheese, and leaner cuts of meat, including pork tenderloin, which has the same amount of total and saturated fat as boneless, skinless chicken breast.

Trans fats: Trans fatty acids are similar to saturated fats in that they, too, are not essential for good health. In fact, studies suggest that increased trans fat intake is linked to a higher risk for cardiovascular disease, in part because trans fat raises LDL cholesterol levels.

There's no need to eat any trans fat, but it's difficult to completely avoid it. Very small amounts of trans fats are found in fatty meats and full-fat dairy foods, but there's far more trans fat in foods with partially hydrogenated fats, such as stick margarine, shortening, French fries, and other fast foods, cookies, donuts, and pastries. The process of hydrogenation, which forces hydrogen into vegetable oils, transforms unsaturated fats into trans fats. Hydrogenated fat is firmer, tastes better, and has a longer shelf life, which is considered ideal for processed foods.

You should eat very little, if any, trans fat. The American Heart Association recommends limiting calories from trans fat to 1% or less of your total intake. That amounts to two grams or less in a 2,000-calorie diet. Two tablespoons of stick margarine, one

☐ Sorting Out Solid Fat

Foods with a high concentration of saturated or trans fats are solid at room temperature and are often called "solid fats." Solid fats are mostly found in animal foods and in foods with hydrogenated fat. Seafood is the exception because its harbors predominantly unsaturated fats, which are usually liquid at room temperature and are referred to as oils.

medium order of fat-food French fries, and one doughnut all contain about two grams of trans fat. Check the Nutrition Facts label for trans fat content of packaged foods, and choose products with no trans fats. Because of a labeling loophole, products that say they have no trans fats may have up to .49 grams per serving, however. Check the ingredient list for hydrogenated or partially hydrogenated fat. That's the only way to really know if there is some trans fat in every serving. Healthy spreads, such as I Can't Believe It's Not Butter!, Country Crock, and Promise Buttery Spread are made without any hydrogenated fat, have no cholesterol, and contain 70% less saturated fat than butter.

> *Because of a labeling loophole, products that say they have no trans fats may have up to .49 grams per serving, however. Check the ingredient list for hydrogenated or partially hydrogenated fat—that's the only way to really know.*

Unsaturated fats: MyPlate and the 2010 Dietary Guidelines encourage monounsaturated and polyunsaturated fats in the diet because they're considered heart healthy. Canola oil, olive oil, and safflower oil are rich in monounsaturated fatty acids, and polyunsaturated acids dominate in soybean, corn, and cottonseed oils, but a combination of unsaturated fats is most commonly found in the oils we tend to use the most every day.

Unsaturated fats called omega-3s are also found in seafood. Fish and shellfish harbor docosohexaenoic acid (DHA) and eicosapentaenoic acid (EPA), two omega-3 fats considered heart healthy because they lower the levels of triglycerides (fat in the blood that contributes to heart disease), reduce the risk of sudden death, heart attack, dangerous abnormal heart rhythms, and stroke in people with cardiovascular disease, slow the buildup of plaque in the arteries that blocks the flow of blood to the heart and brain, and lower blood pressure slightly.

English walnuts and vegetable oils (canola, soybean, flaxseed/linseed, and olive) contain alpha-linolenic acid (ALA), an omega-3 fat that serves as the raw material for making DHA and EPA in the body. On it's own, ALA is not considered as potent as DHA or EPA. In addition, the body converts only a small amount of ALA to DHA and EPA.

Seafood is the best source of DHA and EPA. MyPlate recommends that adults eat 8 ounces of cooked fish weekly to get a variety of nutrients, including omega-3s; pregnant and breastfeeding women should include 8 to 12 ounces of safe fish weekly. Some species of fish carry a higher risk of environmental contamination, such as with methylmercury. (See pages 94-98 for more on seafood safety and the omega-3 content of seafood.)

Omega-3s: Should you supplement?

You don't eat enough fish, neither do your children, and it doesn't look like you'll be eating as much as MyPlate advises any time soon. While food is the preferred way to get nutrients, sometimes it's just not possible, and dietary supplements are necessary to fill in the gap. You don't need big doses of omega-3 supplements to reap benefits. Eating 8 ounces of seafood daily provides, on average, 250 milligrams of EPA and DHA, so look for a supplement that provides about that amount.

Dietary supplements make sense for satisfying the American Heart Association's suggested 1 gram (1,000 mg) daily combination of DHA and EPA for people with diagnosed heart disease. The AHA also recommends 2 to 4 grams (2,000 to 4,000 mg) of EPA plus DHA per day provided as dietary supplements to reduce elevated blood triglycerides and specifies that this amount should be take with a physician's supervision.

If you have a bleeding disorder, discuss taking omega-3 supplements with your doctor. People with allergy or hypersensitivity to fish should avoid fish oil or omega-3 fatty acid products derived from fish.

Fat Facts: Translating Them to the Table

You're aware of the four types of fats in foods, and which ones to avoid, but you're unsure how that translates to what to serve yourself and your family. No worries. Fat recommendations aren't always easy to understand.

For one thing, when MyPlate says fat, it really means oils. Oils isn't an official food group, but oils are important, nonetheless. Oils are fats that are liquid at room temperature, like those used in cooking, including vegetable, canola, and olive oils. Oils come from many different plants.

The monounsaturated and polyunsaturated fats found in fish, nuts, and vegetable oils do not raise LDL ("bad") cholesterol levels in the blood, and oils are cholesterol-free. In addition to the essential fatty acids they contain, oils are the major source of vitamin E in the typical American diet. Vitamin E acts as a cellular bodyguard, warding off damage from free radicals, also known as oxidants.

Here's where the oils group gets confusing. Not all the members of the oils category are actually oils. Some are foods that are naturally rich in oils, including seafood, nuts, olives, and avocados, and others are foods that are made up of mainly oil including mayonnaise, certain salad dressings, and soft (tub or squeeze) margarine with no trans fats.

While unsaturated fat is better for you and your children, that doesn't mean you can douse your salad with dressing or slather your bread with all the healthy spreads you want. When it comes to fat, substitution is the name of the game. The trick is to reduce saturated and trans fat and satisfy the bulk of your fat quotas with oils. Adding healthy fat can actually lead to weight gain when you don't cut back on unhealthy fats at the same time.

How much fat for you and your family?

MyPlate isn't perfect. One of the drawbacks of the symbol is that it fails to convey how much fat to eat on a daily basis. Here's how to figure out fat:

Your daily oil allowance depends on calorie needs. The following chart assumes that people get 30 minutes or less of moderate physical activity every day, in addition to normal daily activities. If you're more active, you can eat more calories, and more oils. For a more personalized approach, visit ChooseMyPlate.gov to determine your calorie intake and find out how much fat you can eat on a daily basis.

Age	Daily Oil Allowance (in teaspoons)
2-3 years	3
4-8 years	4
9-13 years, girls and boys	5
14-18 years, girls	5
14-18 years, boys	6
19-30 years, women	6
31 years and older, women	5
19-30 years, men	7
31 years and older, men	6

Source: ChooseMyPlate.gov

What's Not an Oil

Coconut oil and palm kernel oil don't make it into the oils group, even though they are pourable at room temperature. These so-called tropical oils are so high in saturated fat that MyPlate relegates them to the solid fats group because of the potential problems they pose to good health, including clogging your arteries.

What Counts as a Teaspoon of Oil

Some people get the oil they need from foods, while others could easily consume the recommended allowance by substituting oils for some of the solid fats they eat. The following chart lists fatty foods and the amount of oil in teaspoons they serve up.

Food	Portion size	Amount of oil
Vegetable oils (excluding coconut and palm kernel oils)	1 teaspoon	1 teaspoon
Tub margarine (trans fat free)	1 tablespoon	2½ teaspoons
Mayonnaise	1 tablespoon	2½ teaspoons
Italian dressing	1 tablespoon	1 teaspoon
Thousand Island dressing	1 tablespoon	1¼ teaspoons
Olives, ripe, canned	4 large	½ teaspoon
Avocado	¼ medium	1½ teaspoons
Peanut butter	1 tablespoon	2 teaspoons
Peanuts, dry roasted	1 ounce	3 teaspoons
Mixed nuts, dry roasted	1 ounce	3 teaspoons
Cashews, dry roasted	1 ounce	3 teaspoons
Almonds, dry roasted	1 ounce	3 teaspoons
Pistachios	1 ounce	3 teaspoons
Pecans	1 ounce	3 teaspoons
Hazelnuts, dry roasted	1 ounce	4 teaspoons
Sunflower seeds	1 ounce	3 teaspoons

Source: Adapted from ChooseMyPlate.gov

Dietary Fat and Your Child

You're concerned about your child's weight or maybe you'd like to get a head start on preventing heart disease by reducing the fat in your child's diet. Not so fast.

Younger children need more fat for the calories and the essential fatty acids (EFA) it provides. Insufficient fat in the diet may result in poor growth and development, and coming up short on EFA can cause skin problems and abnormalities in vision and the nervous system.

Children require a greater proportion of their energy as fat. Kids ages one to three years should get between 30% and 40% of their calories from fat and four to eighteen year olds need 25% to 35% of their calories from fat. (Adults over the age of 19 should take in 20% to 35% fat calories.)

☑ What type of milk should kids drink?

Milk products are a major source of nutrition for many children. MyPlate, which applies to everyone over the age of two, recommends serving fat-free and low-fat (1%) milk. Children between the ages of one and two years should drink full-fat milk and eat full-fat yogurt for the calories, fat, and cholesterol they provide.

There's no need to count fat grams or to take pains to restrict fat in a child's diet. When you follow the MyPlate plan, your child will naturally get the healthy fat he needs as part of a balanced diet. Avoid offering "diet" and "fat-free" processed foods designed for adults. It's OK to reduce the amount of foods with added solid fats, including snack chips, crackers, cakes, cookies, and candy, but it's not necessary for children to completely avoid them.

Considering Cholesterol

Cholesterol is a lipid, but it's not a type of fat. It's a waxy substance produced by the liver and found only in animal foods.

You need cholesterol to make vitamin D, to produce hormones, including estrogen and testosterone, construct cell walls, and to make bile, which helps you digest fat. Cholesterol is also part of myelin, the sheath that surrounds and protects nerve cells, allowing them to effectively communicate with each other. Your body manufactures all the cholesterol you need. Cholesterol is calorie-free, so dietary cholesterol doesn't contribute any energy.

Sounds like cholesterol is one beneficial compound. Why the bad reputation? While saturated fat is the main dietary culprit that raises LDL cholesterol, the bad kind that contributes to clogged arteries, cholesterol and trans fat have a hand in that process, too.

Your body may make too much cholesterol, you may eat too much cholesterol, or both, resulting in excessive levels of LDL in your bloodstream. When LDLs are elevated, more cholesterol is dumped on the walls of arteries as part of a process that leads to the formation of plaque. With time, plaque narrows blood vessels and makes them less flexible and resilient. Blocked blood vessels lead to a greater chance for heart attack and stroke and may affect other organs, including your kidneys and digestive tract.

Unless you're a vegan, it's impossible to completely avoid cholesterol. As a rule, foods that are high in saturated fat also tend to be high in cholesterol, with some important exceptions, including:

- *Eggs:* An ordinary large egg contains 185 milligrams of cholesterol and 1.6 grams saturated fat. An Eggland's Best large egg supplies 175 milligrams cholesterol and 1 gram saturated fat.
- *Shrimp:* Shrimp supplies 179 milligrams of cholesterol for three ounces, cooked, but only a trace of saturated fat.

MyPlate does not address daily cholesterol intake, but a lower intake of cholesterol is implied in its recommendations to choose lean protein foods and fat-free and low-fat (1%) milk. The 2010 Dietary Guidelines are more specific about cholesterol. They recommend limiting daily intake to 300 milligrams (mg) for adults.

MyPlate does not address daily cholesterol intake, but a lower intake of cholesterol is implied in its recommendations to choose lean protein foods and fat-free and low-fat (1%) milk. The 2010 Dietary Guidelines are more specific, recommending limiting daily intake to 300 mg for adults.

It's safe to say that many of us do not overdo it when it comes to cholesterol consumption. Adult men are the only group that average more than the suggested limit; they get about 350 mg daily. Women consume only about 240 mg a day.

While dietary cholesterol has been shown to raise LDL cholesterol in some people, the effect of cholesterol is reduced when your saturated fat intake is lowered. Overall, the potentially negative effects of cholesterol you get from food are relatively small compared to those of saturated fat and trans fat. So is all this attention on cholesterol misdirected? Maybe.

Cholesterol is often indicted for the company it keeps. Many favorite American foods, including cheese, pizza, and full-fat milk, contain cholesterol as well as saturated fat. What's puzzling is that the 2010 Dietary Guidelines says that evidence suggests eating one whole egg a day—which provides 185 milligrams of cholesterol, and may cause you to exceed the suggested 300-milligram a day level—does not result in increased blood cholesterol concentrations, and it does not increase the risk of cardiovascular disease in healthy people.

Consuming less than 200 milligrams of cholesterol a day as part of a diet low in saturated fat can help people who are at high risk of cardiovascular disease to lower their chances of developing or worsening the condition.

For many people, there's little reason to count cholesterol, but it's good to be aware of the cholesterol in foods. Choosing foods low in saturated fat most of the time helps you keep cholesterol within the recommended ranges.

Food	Cholesterol (milligrams)
Beef, bottom round, cooked, 3 ounces	84
Soft-serve ice cream, vanilla, ½ cup	81
Ground beef, 80% lean, cooked, 3 ounces	77
Chicken breast, skinless, cooked, 3 ounces	73
Haddock, cooked, 3 ounces	66
Salmon, cooked, 3 ounces	60
Scallops, cooked, 3 ounces	45
Yogurt, full-fat, plain, 1 cup	32
Butter, 1 tablespoon	31
Cheddar cheese, 1 ounce	30
Full-fat milk, 1 cup	24
Reduced-fat milk (2%), 1 cup	20
Yogurt, low-fat, plain, 1 cup	15
Yogurt, fat-free, plain, 1 cup	5
Fat-free milk, 1 cup	4
Mayonnaise, regular, 1 tablespoon	4
Mayonnaise, low-fat, 1 tablespoon	4

Source: USDA

What You Should Know About Fat

There's no question that fat and cholesterol play a role in general and heart health. This chapter provided a lot of details about lipids, which may take some time to digest. If it all seems like too much information, focus on the main messages about fat to get started on eating better. Remember that there's no need for everything you eat to be fat-free or low-fat, because some fat is good for you. Whenever possible, substitute foods rich in heart-healthy unsaturated fats, such as oils, for those with saturated and trans fat, including butter; this approach will naturally curb your cholesterol consumption, too. Your newfound awareness of fat and cholesterol will serve you well when you read the next chapter, which deals with choosing protein-rich foods.

CHAPTER 7

Protein Power on MyPlate

HIGH-PROTEIN WEIGHT LOSS diets go in and out of fashion, but the importance of protein never goes out of style. Protein is a major player in supporting good health. Like carbohydrate and fat, protein provides calories, but that's hardly its strong suit.

Protein helps to hold your body together. It's part of cells, which make up tissues and organs. Without protein, no cell could maintain its structure, or function, for that matter. The enzymes and hormones that drive the chemical reactions that allow you and your children to thrive are also proteins, as are so many other vital compounds that make life possible.

Some people should increase their protein intake, while others need to eat less. Excess calories from any source, including protein, can result weight control problems. To minimize total and saturated fat, MyPlate recommends choosing a variety of lean protein foods. Read on to find out how to harness the power of protein on your plate.

Protein Basics

Food protein and the proteins in your body—cells, enzymes, skin, and other tissues, for example—are composed of amino acids, often referred to as the building blocks of protein.

Your body is capable of producing most of the amino acids it needs, but nine of them are classified as "essential" because the body cannot make them. That's where food comes in.

Food protein provides amino acids, including the essential ones, that you need to build body proteins. You must get essential amino acids from foods and beverages. That's why it's important to include enough protein in your eating plan, and your family's.

Food protein provides amino acids, including the essential ones, that you need to build body proteins. You must get essential amino acids from foods and beverages. That's why it's important to include enough protein in your eating plan, and your family's.

The Possibilities of Protein on Your Plate

MyPlate groups all meat, poultry, seafood, beans, peas, eggs, soy products, nuts, and seeds into the proteins food group, formerly known as the meat and beans group. While the members of this category have protein in common, their differences matter, too.

Whether you're a mainstream eater, a vegetatarian, or a "flexitarian," someone who eats meat and seafood occasionally, including an array of protein-rich foods in a balanced eating plan improves your nutrient intake and provides other benefits, too. See what other nutrients protein-rich foods include:

- Dairy foods contain bone-building calcium.
- Nuts, such as almonds, supply significant amounts of vitamin E, and they supply an array of other nutrients.
- Soy products contain potent, protective phytotnutrients, plant compounds that guard against cell damage.
- Meat, poultry, and pork provide iron and zinc.
- Seafood supplies heart-healthy omega-3 fats. MyPlate suggests adults eat at least 8 ounces of cooked seafood a week. This recommendation does not apply to people who don't eat animal foods, and children need less fish than adults.
- Beans and peas supply fiber and provide iron and zinc in amounts similar to seafood, meat, and poultry.

In an effort to direct people toward a more plant-based diet, the government's lastest food guidance program recommends replacing some meat and poultry with legumes, nuts, and seeds, such sunflower, sesame, and pumpkin. Nuts and seeds are relatively high in calories and heart-healthy fat for the protein they provide, so it's unreasonable to expect to satisfy most of your daily protein needs with nuts and seeds because you would likely exceed your calorie budget in doing so.

◻ Go Nuts for Heart Health!

Eating just 1½ ounces of tree nuts, such as walnuts, almonds, and pistachios, or peanuts, daily as part of a low-cholesterol, low-saturated-fat eating plan may reduce your risk for heart disease. Use nuts to replace other protein foods rather than adding them to what you already eat to avoid excess calories, and choose unsalted nuts.

Choose Protein, Not Fat

In addition to including a variety of protein-packed foods, the 2010 Dietary Guidelines and MyPlate recommend opting for choices with the least solid fats.

Solid fat, which is often highly-saturated fat, contributes to clogged arteries. Fat found in animal foods such as meat, poultry, and cheese is considered solid fat, while the fats found in seafood, nuts, and seeds are classified as oils. Oils are heart-healthy fats.

The typical American eating pattern is rife with solid fat. Solid fats, found naturally in foods and added to processed products, can add hundreds of calories every day that may contribute to weight management problems.

Cutting back on fat doesn't necessarily mean dining on fat-free and low-fat foods at every meal and snack, however. It's possible to balance higher-fat protein foods, including marbled cuts of beef and full-fat cheese, with lower-fat protein-packed options, such as fat-free and low-fat (1%) milk and yogurt, low-fat cottage cheese, beans, and certain soy products.

How much protein for you and your family?
The amount of protein you need every day is linked to your calorie needs. Adults and teens require about 6½-ounce equivalents of protein foods daily. Younger children should eat between 2 and 5 ounces as part of a balanced diet that also includes the recommended servings of dairy foods, which help to satisfy protein needs.

What's an ounce equivalent? It's the amount of food equal to 1 ounce of meat, poultry, or seafood. For example, an egg is an ounce equivalent. Here are some more MyPlate food group examples of what counts as an ounce of protein:

- 1 ounce cooked meat, poultry, or fish or 1 ounce cooked deli meat, such as turkey
- ¼ cup cooked beans or peas, such as black, kidney, and garbanzo bean, or lentils
- 1 tablespoon peanut butter or almond butter
- ½ ounce of nuts (12 almonds, 24 pistachios, 7 walnut halves)
- ¼ cup tofu (about 2 ounces)
- 1 ounce cooked tempeh
- ½ cup roasted soybeans
- 2 tablespoons hummus
- ½ cup split pea, lentil, or bean soup

Source: ChooseMyPlate.gov

Another Way to Figure Protein Needs

There's more than one way to find out how much protein you need every day. It's not necessary to count every gram of protein you eat, but you may be interested in checking out your eating pattern every once in a while to see if you're including the protein you need. Teenage girls and women may not be getting the protein they need. The protein guidelines below, and the chart that follows, will alert you to insufficiencies or excesses in your diet.

Age	Daily protein needs (in grams)
1-3 years	13
4-8 years	19
9-13 years	34
14-18 years, female	46
14-18 years, male	52
19 years and older, female	46
19-30 years and older, male	46
Pregnant or nursing	71

Source: IOM

Now that you know your daily protein goals, use the chart below to determine if you're getting enough protein from a variety of foods, most of which are low in solid fats.

Food	Protein (grams)
Chicken breast, skinless, cooked, 3 ounces	26
Pork tenderloin, cooked, 3 ounces	22
Beef, 95% lean, roasted, 3 ounces	22
Salmon, Atlantic, cooked, 3 ounces	22
Tuna, light, canned, drained, 3 ounces	22
Shrimp, cooked, 3 ounces	19
Greek yogurt, plain, fat-free, 6 ounces	18
Greek yogurt, fruit, fat-free, 6 ounces	14
Cottage cheese, low-fat, ½ cup	13
Yogurt, plain, low-fat, 1 cup	13
Tofu, raw, ½ cup	10
Peanut butter, 2 tablespoons	9
Milk, full-fat or 1% low-fat, 1 cup	8
Lentils, cooked, ½ cup	8
Black beans, canned, drained, ½ cup	7
Cheddar cheese, 1 ounce	7

Food	Protein (grams)
Soy beverage, 1 cup	7
Almonds, roasted, 1 ounce	6
Egg, raw or cooked, large	6
Pistachios, shelled, 1 ounce	6
Garbanzo beans, canned, drained, ½ cup	6
Walnuts, shelled, 1 ounce	4

Source: USDA

Eggs

Eggs supply the highest-quality protein of any food, and egg protein is used as the standard for comparing all other food proteins for their ability to promote and sustain life.

If you've been avoiding eggs out of concerns about cholesterol, you can stop now. Most healthy people can eat an egg a day as part of a balanced low-fat diet without raising their risk for heart disease. People with diabetes may need to eat fewer eggs and should talk to their registered dietitian or doctor about what's right for them.

Eggs supply choline, a nutrient also found in many other members in the protein foods group. Choline is an essential nutrient that plays a key role in the development of the part of the brain responsible for memory functions during pregnancy, and may also head off certain birth defects. The egg yolk contains choline, all the other vitamins and minerals that eggs provide, and about half the protein.

Fortified eggs are better for you than regular eggs. For example, Eggland's Best eggs provide 10 times the vitamin E of ordinary eggs, twice as much of vitamins A and D, 75% more vitamin B12, and double the docosahexaenoic acid (DHA), a beneficial omega-3 fat, and they have just 175 milligrams of cholesterol, and 25% less saturated fat than regular eggs.

Go Fishing for Good Nutrition

MyPlate recommends a variety of protein foods, but seafood gets special attention. Swap some seafood for meat and poultry for a total intake of at least 8 ounces a week for adults; pregnant and nursing women are advised to put 8 to 12 ounces of seafood on their plates every week.

As recommendations go, suggesting seafood instead of meat and poultry is a first in the history of the government's eating advice.

Considering our current seafood consumption, it may be a bit of a stretch to achieve the suggested amount on a regular basis. The average American consumes about 3½ ounces of fish a week; pregnant women include less than two ounces weekly. Yet, while most of us have a long way to go to meet the 8-ounce weekly minimum for seafood, it's a worthy pursuit.

In addition to protein, seafood harbors iron, selenium, and potassium, and it's relatively low in cholesterol. Seafood is also an important source of the omega-3 fats, eicosapentaenoic acid (EPA) and DHA. Eight ounces of a variety of seafood weekly provides an estimated average of 250 milligrams (mg) of EPA and DHA a day, an amount associated with a lower risk of death from heart disease among healthy people. Omega-3 fats, particularly DHA, are linked to brain development and peak vision during pregnancy and early childhood.

☐ Seafood, Defined

Seafood comes from the sea, right? Not exactly. The 2010 Dietary Guidelines define seafood as marine animals that live in the sea and in freshwater lakes and rivers. Seafood includes all fish, and shellfish, such as shrimp, crab, and oysters.

Seafood Safety

If you're of childbearing age and are capable of becoming pregnant, or you're pregnant or breastfeeding, eating seafood is a good idea, as long as that seafood is on the safe side. The level of methylmercury in seafood is the main safety concern for women capable of having children.

When mercury is emitted into the atmosphere by coal-burning power plants and by other industrial activities, it eventually lands in the bodies of water where fish and shellfish live. The bacteria in oceans, lakes, ponds, and streams convert mercury into methylmercury, the most dangerous form of this heavy metal. When fish eat plants and smaller fish with mercury, they get a dose of methylmercury. Larger fish tend to have the highest methylmercury levels because they are older and have had more time to accumulate mercury in their flesh.

Methlymercury builds up in our bodies, too, and it's possible to pass it to your unborn child during pregnancy and when nursing. Methylmercury is harmful to the brain and nervous system and causes irreversible damage.

The U.S. Food and Drug Administration (FDA) warns women against eating the following higher-mercury fish during their child-bearing years to reduce the risk to themselves and their children:

- tilefish
- shark
- swordfish
- king mackerel

Searching for Safer Seafood

You may find feel like your drowning in seafood advice, but don't let the recommendations about safer seafood scare you off this nutrient-rich protein source. Overall, research suggests that the benefits of eating seafood far outweigh the potential risks.

Including a wide variety of smaller fish, including shrimp, tilapia, oysters, sardines, and salmon greatly reduces the risk of mercury consumption. The FDA says canned light tuna, salmon, Pollock, and catfish are five of the most commonly eaten fish that are low in mercury, and considered safe for women in their child-bearing years.

What about canned white tuna, another Ameri-can favorite? Women in their childbearing years don't need to avoid canned white tuna, but they should limit it to six ounces a week, as part of the 12 ounces of seafood they're advised to eat. The FDA does not include other forms of tuna in their advisory, but as you can see in the chart on the following page, bluefin, skipjack, and yellowfin are among the fish highest in mercury.

Women in their child-bearing years don't need to avoid canned white tuna, but they should limit it to six ounces a week, as part of the 12 ounces of seafood they're advised to eat.

You'll gain the greatest benefits from seafood with the highest levels of omega-3 fats and the lowest concentrations of mercury. You don't need to count every milligram (mg) of omega-3 fat that passes your lips, but in case you're wondering how much you need, the Dietary Guidelines recommend at least 1,750 mg of EPA and DHA combined (an average of 250 mg/day), every week.

Here is a list of low-mercury seafood that's also rich in omega-3 fats:

Seafood, 4 ounces, cooked	Mercury (mcg)	EPA + DHA (mg)
Shrimp	0	100
Clams	0	200-300
Tilapia	2	150
Salmon: Atlantic, Chinook, Coho	2	1,200-2,400
Salmon: Pink and Sockeye	2	700-900
Oysters: Pacific	2	1,550
Sardines: Atlantic and Pacific	2	1,100-1,600
Haddock and Hake	2-5	200
Crayfish	5	200
Anchovies, Herring, and Shad	5-10	2,300-2,400
Pollock: Atlantic and Walleye	6	600
Catfish	7	100-250
Flounder, Plaice, Sole	7	350
Scallops	8	200
Mackerel: Atlantic and Pacific (not King*)	8-13	1,350-2,100
Crab: Blue, King, Snow, Queen, Dungeness	9	200-550
Trout: Freshwater	11	1,000-1,100
Tuna, light canned	13	150-300
Cod: Atlantic and Pacific	14	200
Lobsters: Northern, American	47	200

These varieties of seafood are among the highest in mercury content:

Seafood, 4 ounces, cooked	Mercury (mcg)	EPA + DHA (mg)
Tuna: Bluefin, Albacore	54-58	1700
Tuna: White (Albcacore) canned	40	1,000
Tuna: Skipjack and Yellowfin	31-49	150-350
Lobsters: Northern, American	47	200
Shark*	151	1250
Tilefish*	219	1000
Swordfish*	147	1000
Mackerel: King*	110	450

Women in their childbearing years and young children should not eat these fish.
Source: Dietary Guidelines for Americans, 2010, Appendix 11

How much seafood for kids?

Young children should follow the same recommendations as women in their reproductive years about what fish to completely avoid, and should eat low-mercury fish and shellfish, too.

Young children have lower calorie requirements, so feed them less fish. Two to three-year-olds need about 1,000 calories a day; three to four year olds need between 1,000 calories and 1,400 daily, depending on their activity level; pre-teens need about 1,400 to 1,600 calories each day. Use these requirements with the following seafood guidelines for children.

Here are some examples of how much seafood the Dietary Guidelines recommend on a weekly basis for children:

Daily Calorie Needs	Suggested Seafood Intake/Week (cooked)
1,000	3 ounces
1,200	5 ounces
1,400	6 ounces
1,600	8 ounces

 ## How to Eat More Seafood

Some people don't like fish, period. Others are allergic to seafood and must avoid it. However, you may want to eat more seafood. Here's how to overcome the most common obstacles to putting seafood on MyPlate.

- **You don't know how to prepare it.** Other than making tuna fish sandwiches and adding canned salmon to salads, you're lost when it comes to making delicious seafood dishes. See chapter 9 for family-friendly seafood recipes. If you don't care to cook it, order seafood when you dine out to work more into your diet.

- **You think seafood is expensive.** Seafood can be one of the more expensive protein sources. Wild salmon may taste great, but it's just not in the family food budget. No worries. Get the most for your food dollars by choosing seafood that harbors the most omega-3 fats, and keeping portions with the recommended amount. Stretch seafood by using it in salads, casseroles, tacos, sandwiches, pasta dishes, and soups. Buy seafood on sale to save money, too.

- **You think seafood tastes too strong.** Try milder-tasting fish, including tilapia, farmed catfish, cod, flounder, haddock, and shrimp.

More tips next page...

...Continued from previous page

- **You think seafood is inconvenient.** Seafood is one of the most convenient and versatile protein foods. You can easily grill or broil fish and serve it with salsa or another easy sauce. Tuna and salmon are available in pouches, and clams and shrimp come in cans, too. Try seasoned single-serve cans of tuna for lunch or a snack. It's portable and ready to make a meal along with a whole-wheat roll and fruit. Rely on frozen fish burgers and frozen shrimp for quick meals, too.

- **You're concerned about sustainability.** According to the Monterey Bay Aquarium's Seafood Watch, some of the most sustainable and environmentally-friendly fish to eat include wild Alaskan salmon, farmed Arctic char, and U.S.-farmed shrimp and catfish. For more on seafood sustainability, visit the Monterey Bay Aquarium at www.montereybayaquarium.org/cr/seafoodwatch.aspx

Vegetarian and Vegan Eating Plans: Get the Nutrients You Need

In general, animal products, such as meat, eggs, poultry, seafood, and dairy, supply all the essential amino acids you need, as long as you eat the right amount of protein foods every day. With the exception of soy, plant foods lack one or more of the essential amino acids.

Vegetarians and vegans—people who avoid all animal products—should include an array of protein-rich plant foods, including beans and soy products, as part of a balanced diet. Vegans may be at risk for low intakes of several nutrients, including iron, choline, omega-3 fats, vitamins B12 and D, and calcium, so it's important to choose fortified products, such as soy beverages with added calcium and vitamin D, to get the nutrients missing from animal foods.

If you include dairy and eggs in your diet, the risk of low intake of several nutrients decreases, but the concern about iron remains. No matter what type of eater you are, it's important to consume the level of protein that's right for you every day. In addition, taking a multivitamin helps to fill in small nutrient gaps, and is especially useful for satisfying iron requirements.

The Bottom Line on Protein

Here's the least you need to know about protein. It's paramount for good health, especially in children, whether you're a vegetarian, mainstream eater, or flexitarian. With protein, variety is the name of the game, and it's possible to get the protein you need with any number of protein-rich foods. Lastly, lower-fat animal and plant foods should dominate your protein choices, no matter what your age or stage of life.

CHAPTER 8

Rethink Your Drink

AN ENTIRE CHAPTER devoted to beverages? It makes sense when you consider that our drinking habits are making it difficult to achieve a healthy weight and maintain it. In fact, two out of 10 My-Plate messages are devoted to what to drink.

If you're like most adults and children, you guzzle hundreds of calories a day with little nutrition to show for it. Alcoholic beverages supply a steady stream of calories for adults, while popular coffee and energy drinks that are dripping with caffeine can play havoc with your health, and your child's.

Don't despair—there's no need to sip only plain water, give up your daily glass of wine, or pass on your favorite coffee-shop beverage. But it does pay to consider which drinks are worthy of your precious calories, and which ones are waistline-wreckers.

Liquid Sugar

Taken together, soda, energy beverages, sports drinks, and sugar-sweetened fruit concoctions account for a whopping 46% of the calories we consume from added sugars.

This may sound strange, but cookies, cake, and other confections are not the top sources of added sugar in the American diet. Sugary beverages have that honor, and by far outpace the contribution of added sugars from other foods.

Taken together, soda, energy beverages, sports drinks, and sugar-sweetened fruit concoctions account for a whopping 46% of the calories we consume from added sugars. And that's not counting the sugar we stir into our coffee and tea.

Some of us are drinking ourselves overweight. Of course, sipping sugary beverages isn't the sole reason for the calorie imbalance that leads to weight gain, but it's certainly easier to guzzle calories that don't seem to contribute to feelings of fullness. People seldom reduce their food intake to accommodate the calories they drink. The result is excess energy, which is particularly problematic in children.

How much sugar is OK every day?

MyPlate and the 2010 Dietary Guidelines for Americans don't provide exact guidelines for added sugars, but the American Heart Association (AHA) gets more specific about daily sugar intake.

The AHA recommends spending no more than half of the calories you're allowed every day for added fats and sugars after you've selected the suggested amounts of low-fat and fat-free dairy, lean protein foods, grains, and fruits and vegetables. In the past, this "bank" of calories was referred to as Discretionary Calories, which you can think of as calories to spend how you want. In the 2010 version of the dietary guidelines, this category of calories is called Maximum SoFAS. (SoFAS stand for calories from solid fats and added sugars.)

Here's a chart that makes the AHA's guidelines more clear for a variety of calorie levels. Calorie levels are daily goals, and sugar limits are provided in teaspoons with the equivalent is given in grams to help make reading food labels easier. Daily sugar limits do not apply to foods that are naturally sweet, such as 100% fruit juice and fruit. Nor do they apply to milk and yogurt, which contain lactose. Lactose is a naturally occurring sugar which must be listed as such on the food label. Lactose is not added sugar.

Daily Calorie Intake	SoFAS Calorie Limit	Daily Sugar Limit
1,400	121	4 teaspoons; 16 grams
1,600	121	4 teaspoons; 16 grams
1,800	161	5 teaspoons; 20 grams
2,000	258	8 teaspoons; 32 grams
2,200	266	8 teaspoons; 32 grams
2,400	330	10 teaspoons; 40 grams
3,000	459	14 teaspoons; 57 grams

Source: American Heart Association

For some perspective on how much sugar beverages supply, check out some of the top sugar contributors.

Drink	Sugar (in level teaspoons)
Carbonated soft drink, 12 ounces	9 to 12
Sports drink, 16 ounces	8
Energy drink, 8.3 ounces	7
Lemonade, 8 ounces	7

Source: USDA

The Juicy Details

Juice supplies sugar, but it's a worthy beverage choice; 100% fruit juice derives its sweetness from naturally-occurring sugars. Nutritionally speaking, 100% fruit juice is head and shoulders above juice beverages, soda, energy drinks, and sports drinks.

Juice supplies minerals, including potassium, a nutrient that often comes up short in the typical American diet; vitamins, such as vitamin C; and phytonutrients, disease-fighting plant compounds. Juice may also be fortified with vitamins, including vitamin D, and calcium, adding to its nutritional arsenal. However, juice lacks the fiber found in whole fruit, and it is possible to drink too much.

Juice is a great way to work in more fruit, which the Dietary Guidelines recommend. Kids favor juice more than adults, and experts recommend limits on their intake.

The American Academy of Pediatrics suggests waiting until at least six months to introduce juice to infants, and capping daily juice consumption to six ounces (3/4 cup) a day until the age of six. Never fill a baby's bottle with juice. Kids may become accustomed to the juice and refuse the more nutritious breast milk or infant formula they need to grow and develop properly. In addition, the high natural sugar levels in juice can cause diarrhea, even in healthy children.

Juice is a great way to work in more fruit, which the Dietary Guidelines recommend. Kids favor juice more than adults, and experts recommend limits on their intake.

When choosing juice, always pick 100% fruit juice. You'll find the percentage of fruit juice at the top of the Nutrition Facts Panel on food packages. Avoid juice concoctions with the terms "cocktail" or "-ade" (as in lemonade); they contain less than 100% juice and many are nothing more than sugar-flavored water. Opt for brands that offer added nutrients, such as vitamin D or calcium, or both. Drink only pasteurized juice to reduce the chance of illness from germs. The label will specify whether the product is pasteurized.

Count Your Cocktails

You may dream of a drink at the end of a day, after a long week at work, or on a night out. Moderate alcohol intake, defined by the Dietary Guidelines as up to one drink daily for women and up to two a day for men, may offer some health benefits. Boozy beverages probably won't interfere with weight control, as long as you account for the calories they contain. Measuring alcoholic drinks will help you track your calories and adhere to the guidelines for daily alcohol limits.

One drink is defined by the 2010 Dietary Guidelines as:
- 12 ounces of regular beer (5% alcohol), or
- 5 ounces of wine (12% alcohol), or
- 1.5 ounces of 80-proof distilled spirits, such as vodka, rum, or gin

Calculating Alcohol Calories
Wine and other spirits have plenty of calories. When combined with mixers like full-fat milk, cream, fruit juice, soda, and others, the calories in alcoholic beverages can easily double, triple, or more, turning your reasonable drink into a significant source of added sugar, added fat, or both.

With the words "caramel" or "chocolate" in drink names, some concoctions should be considered dessert in a glass. Mixed drinks are exceptionally caloric, unless the mixer is seltzer water, calorie-free tonic water, water, a diet soft drink, club soda, or some other calorie-free fluid.

Beverage	Calories
Mud slide, 4 ounces	520
Chocolate martini, 4 ounces	438
Cosmopolitan, 3 ounces	220
Vodka and tonic, 4 ounces	178
Rum and cola, 4 ounces	178
53-proof coffee liquor, 1.5 ounces	170
Caramel Appeltini, 3 ounces	160
Regular beer, 12 ounces	150
Screwdriver, with light orange juice	146
Bloody Mary, 4 ounces	146
Wine, including Champagne and sparkling wine, 5 ounces	121
Hard iced tea, 12 ounces	115
80-proof rum, gin, vodka, or whiskey, 1.5 ounces	96
Rum and diet cola, 4 ounces	96
Gin and diet tonic water, 4 ounces	96
Light beer, 12 ounces	64-110
Wine spritzer, 4 ounces	48

Source: USDA

The Pros and Cons of Alcohol

Other than calories (seven per gram, nearly twice that of carbohydrate and protein), alcohol offers no nutrients. Alcohol can spell disaster for healthy eating by lowering inhibitions and lessening your resolve to eat right, which may result in overdoing it on food at restaurants. Yet, drinking may support good health for other reasons.

Some studies show that moderate drinking is linked to a lower risk of cardiovascular disease, a reduced risk of death from any cause during middle-age, and better brain function with age. Avoiding alcohol also lowers blood pressure, especially in combination with a healthy diet and regular physical activity. There's no need to begin drinking or to drink more frequently to get these benefits, however. If you don't drink already, don't start.

The downside is that moderate alcohol intake is also associated with an increased risk of breast cancer, violence, drowning, and injuries from falls and motor vehicle crashes.

Some People Should Not Drink

Certain people should avoid alcohol completely, according to 2010 Dietary Guidelines and other experts, including the following:

- Those who are unable to restrict their drinking to moderate levels.
- Anyone under the legal drinking age.
- Pregnant women or those who may be pregnant. There is no known safe level of alcohol intake when you're expecting a child.
- People taking medication, including over-the-counter drugs, that interact with alcohol. Ask your pharmacist if you're in doubt.
- People with certain medical conditions, including liver disease.
- Those who plan to drive, operate machinery, or take part in any other activity that requires coordination and concentration or in situations where impaired judgment could cause injury or death.

 ## Easy Ways to Cut Back on Alcohol

- **Decrease alcohol intake by half, to start.** For example, sip a wine spritzer made with two ounces wine instead of a five-ounce glass of wine every day and save 26,280 calories in a year's time, the equivalent of about 7.5 pounds of body fat.
- **Don't refill your glass before it's empty.** You'll lose track of how much you've had to drink.
- **Always begin with a calorie-free nonalcoholic beverage** and alternate that type of drink with an alcoholic drink.
- **When you're dining out, wait until the meal arrives** to have an alcoholic beverage. Eating slows alcohol intake and food reduces alcohol absorption in the body.

Out of Control Alcohol

Heavy drinking, also known as high-risk drinking, is downing more than three drinks on any day and more than seven drinks a week for women, according to the Dietary Guidelines. For men, heavy drinking is considered having more than four drinks on any day, or more than 14 a week. An episode of binge drinking is consuming four drinks or more within two hours for women, and five or more drinks within the same time span for men.

Any type of excessive alcohol intake presents far more health hazards than moderate drinking, and has no known benefits. Over time, excessive drinking promotes weight gain and is capable of

Alcohol Advice for Breastfeeding Moms

Alcohol gets into breast milk and may slow the development of your child's motor skills, which influence activities such as walking and grabbing large objects. You don't necessarily need to give up alcohol as a nursing mom, however. The 2010 Dietary Guidelines suggests waiting until three months after delivery to drink if you're a nursing mom. To reduce the chances of passing alcohol to your baby, enjoy a single alcoholic beverage four hours before breast-feeding. You can also express breast milk before having a drink and feed the baby by bottle with that milk later.

impairing your day-to-day thinking and reasoning skills. It also increases the risk of liver disease, high blood pressure, stroke, type 2 diabetes, cancer of the upper digestive tract and colon, injury, and violence.

Water

Water is an underappreciated nutrient. That's right, water is a nutrient. When water is in short supply, it will kill you faster than any other nutrient deficiency. What's more, water is an *essential* nutrient, which means the body cannot make water, and must get it from an outside source.

The body is 60% to 75% water, depending on your age and gender. Children have a higher water content than older people, and men carry around more water than women.

Water is working for you all the time to keep your body running smoothly. Here's what water does:

- *Acts as a solvent.* Water dissolves certain nutrients, such as the B vitamins and vitamin C, allowing them to reach your cells.
- *Prevents overheating.* A bodily temperature of about 98.6° F is ideal for life-giving processes. Water helps to maintain that optimum temperature in part by allowing us to sweat, which helps the body get rid of the heat generated by everyday metabolism and physical activity. You sweat 24/7, although it's more noticeable during hot and humid weather.
- *Protects joints and internal organs.* Water is necessary to help joints move and to protect them, and to cushion your internal organs.

- *Aids in transportation.* Water is part of fluids, such as blood, that ferry nutrients to cells, and carts away waste products.
- *Maintains fluid balance.* Blood is about 83% water. The body needs water to keep blood volume in check, which affects circulation and overall health.
- *Lubricates.* Water is part of the mucous and salivary juices in the digestive system, where it helps move food through the digestion process.
- *Forms urine.* Water is the basis of urine, which carries waste products from the body. Without urine, your body would quickly turn toxic.

▣ Full of Fluid

MyPlate recommends filling half your plate with fruits and vegetables for the nutrients they provide, including fluid. Fruits and vegetable are bursting with water, while fattier foods have only small amounts; one cup of cubed watermelon supplies nearly five ounces of water and a medium apple contains nearly three ounces.

How much fluid for you?

"Let thirst be your guide" is a good way to gauge how much fluid you need. Generally speaking, younger children, ages one to eight, require about four to five 8-ounce cups of water daily; kids from nine to 18 need about 8 to 11 cups; women who are not pregnant or nursing, 9 cups; and adult men, 13 cups a day. Pregnant women should aim for 10 cups of fluid daily, while breastfeeding moms need about thirteen 8-ounce cups, as water is the basis of breast milk.

Active people and those who work outside in a warm environment probably need more water. Most active people do not need sports drinks, which can contribute extra calories. Generally speaking, sports drinks are useful only when working out continuously in a vigorous fashion, like running or biking, for 60 minutes or more in a vigorous fashion.

MyPlate recommends drinking water instead of sugary drinks for Americans of all ages. Plain water is preferable for fulfilling fluid needs, but the water in other fluids, such as fat-free and low-fat (1%) milk, 100% juice, coffee, tea, and other soft drinks go toward your daily water needs, too. According to the Institute of Medicine, caffeinated beverages can be part of your daily total fluid intake.

However, too much caffeine can cause problems. See more on caffeine, below. As for alcohol, while it promotes some water loss from the body, losses are not considered significant with moderate drinking, so alcohol counts toward fluid intake.

The Caffeine Conundrum

As anyone knows who stumbles to the kitchen when they get out of bed in the morning in search of coffee, or who experiences a mid-afternoon energy slump, caffeine is a stimulant that revs up the central nervous system, increasing alertness.

While a little caffeine provides the jolt you need, too much can leave you jittery during the day and unable to sleep soundly at night, which, ironically, may result in even greater caffeine consumption during your waking hours. Excess caffeine may also be the source of headaches.

Caffeine is considered a diuretic-a substance that promotes urination-but it's unclear if caffeine causes dehydration because its effects are generally considered as fleeting, and probably don't affect those who are well-hydrated.

Most healthy people can tolerate small quantities of caffeine without problems, but caffeine isn't entirely in the clear. Caffeine can aggravate certain heart conditions, such as an abnormal heart rhythm, and it's capable of interacting with medications and dietary supplements. Stressed and anxious people may find that caffeine heightens these emotions.

Caffeine can aggravate certain heart conditions, such as an abnormal heart rhythm, and it's capable of interacting with medications and dietary supplements.

Experts say caffeine may also cause bone tissue loss, but high caffeine consumption may only be problematic when your diet is also low in calcium. Caffeine-containing soft drinks and coffee often replace fat-free and low-fat (1%) milk, causing a shortage of calcium in the diet and a possible excess of caffeine. Adequate calcium intake offers protection against any possible effects of caffeine on bones.

How much caffeine is OK every day? There are no exact daily limits from the U.S. government, but Health Canada, the Canadian government's agency responsible for helping Canadians maintain and improve their health, says that the general population of healthy adults is at no risk for unhealthy effects from caffeine at 400 milligrams (mg) a day or less.

Women in their childbearing years should consume not more than 300 mg of caffeine a day, according to Health Canada, while the March of Dimes recommends a limit of 200 mg. Caffeine intake has been linked to a greater risk of miscarriage, but the research is inconclusive. Still, it's safe to err on the side of caution when you're pregnant, or trying for a child. See the chart below and on the following page for how many milligrams of caffeine are in common foods and beverages.

Kids and Caffeine

There's no agreement on how much caffeine American kids are consuming, but it's safe to say that children are sipping more caffeinated coffee, soft drinks, and energy beverages than ever.

Kids are smaller than adults and tend to experience a heightened reaction to the stimulant effects of caffeine. As a result, caffeine is more inclined to produce anxiety, headache, and poor sleep in kids. The United States Food and Drug Administration has not developed caffeine guidelines (maximum suggested daily intake) for children. Here are the suggested daily limits from Health Canada:

- Ages 4 to 6: 45 mg
- Ages 7 to 9: 62.5 mg
- Ages 10 to 12: 85 mg

There are no definitive guidelines for kids 13 years and older from Health Canada, but the agency suggests no more than 2.5 milligrams of caffeine per kilogram (a kilogram is equal to 2.2 pounds) of body weight or 1.3 mg for every pound. For example, a child who weighs 100 pounds should limit daily caffeine intake to 113 mg.

Java Jolt!

Caffeine is prevalent in coffee and coffee drinks, but it's also found in a number of other foods. Find out how much caffeine you and your kids consume.

Food or Beverage	Caffeine (mg)
FIXX Extreme, 1 packet	400
Starbucks Brewed Coffee (Grande), 16 ounces	330
Spike Shooter, 8.4 ounces	300
Einstein Bros. regular coffee, 16 ounces	300
Starbucks Iced Brewed coffee, 16 ounces	190
Monster Energy, 16 ounces	160

Food or Beverage	Caffeine (mg)
Foosh Energy Mints, 1 piece	100
Coffee, generic brewed, 8 ounces	95
SoBe No Fear, 8 ounces	87
Red Bull, 8.3 ounce	75
Starbucks Espresso, solio, 1 ounce	75
Jolt Cola, 12 ounces	72
Mountain Dew, regular or diet, 12 ounces	54
Diet Coke, 12 ounces	47
Tea, black, brewed, 8 ounces	47
Aquafina Alive Energize, 8 ounces	46
Snapple, Lemon Iced Teas, regular and diet, 16 ounces	42
Arizona Iced Tea, black, 20 ounces	31

Source: Manufacturer data

Make the Most of Milk

MyPlate recommends drinking fat-free and low-fat (1%) milk and fortified soy beverages. Dairy foods offer an array of nutrients, and milk is particularly rich in three of the four nutrients identified as lacking in our diets: calcium, vitamin D, and potassium. Milk is also a substantial source of protein, B vitamins, vitamin A, and phosphorus.

Lower-fat milk appears to be so popular that it may seem strange that people drink more whole milk and 2% reduced-fat milk than the even lower-fat kinds. Any type of milk is good for you, but whole milk and 2% reduced-fat milk are sources of solid fats, contributing more saturated fat and calories to your diet than their lower-fat counterparts, and more cholesterol, too.

When you make the switch to lower-fat milk, you cut calories, fat, and cholesterol, but you don't compromise good nutrition. That's because the levels of other nutrients in milk are the same in fat-free, low-fat (1%), and flavored milks as they are in whole milk and 2% reduced-fat milk.

When you make the switch to lower-fat milk, you cut calories, fat, and cholesterol, but you don't compromise good nutrition.

Drink It In

As you can see, there's really no point in wasting calories on drinks when you could be spending them on food. In addition, your choice of beverages plays a big role in helping you to get the nutrients you need, and avoiding the ones you don't. This is especially true for children, who have a tendency to fill up on fluids and not have room for more nutritious foods. Getting into the habit of drinking only the most nutritious beverages is a step toward a healthier diet, and the sooner that happens, the better. Choosing water, milk, and 100% juice is an easy change that everyone in the family can make, starting now.

CHAPTER 9

Now You're Cooking! MyPlate Meals and Snacks

MYPLATE provides the blueprint for good health by reminding you about making nutritious food choices that fit with your calorie needs. But all the nutrition information in the world won't do much good unless you know how to translate it to what foods to put on your plate, in your hand, or in your glass.

When it comes right down to it, busy people need simple solutions for eating better. You want the basics of putting together nutritious and delicious meals and snacks, without the fuss. Before you rush to the kitchen, consider food safety, a subject the 2010 Dietary Guidelines for Americans take seriously.

Keep Foods Safe: The Basics

You're eager to know what to feed yourself and your family. But first, a few words about food safety.

Preventing foodborne illness is central to good health. You can't control what happens to your food before you buy it, but there are several steps to take at home to reduce your risk of getting sick. Here are the four basic principles of safe food handling that you should make part of your routine.

◻ Meals Matter, But Patterns Prevail

MyPlate promotes healthy food choices at every meal and snack, yet no single meal or snack makes or breaks your diet. It's your overall eating habits that matter most. The Dietary Guidelines refer to several ways of eating as being particularly good for you, which is good news for mainstream eaters, vegetarians, vegans, and others.

Clean

- Before you handle any food, wash your hands with warm soapy water for at least 20 seconds.
- When you can't use soap, rely on alcohol-based gel formulas or wipes.
- Wash all the produce you eat thoroughly. Use a small vegetable brush to remove dirt from thick or rough-skinned fruits and vegetables.
- Clean cutting boards, dishes, utensils, and countertops thoroughly with dishwashing soap or a cleaning agent.

Separate

- Separate ready-to-eat foods, such as salad greens, from raw animal foods.
- Use separate cutting boards for raw foods, and separate plates for raw and cooked foods.
- Wash your hands after handling raw meat, poultry, seafood, or eggs and before touching ready-to-eat foods.

Cook and Chill

- Keep your refrigerator at 40°F and your freezer at 0°F or below. Monitor temperatures with an appliance thermometer.
- You can't tell if a food is properly cooked by the way it looks. Always use a food thermometer to test the doneness of seafood, meat, poultry, and egg dishes. Visit www.isitdoneyet.gov for proper temperatures.
- Refrigerate foods after two hours; one hour if the air temperature is 90°F or above. This applies to time spent grocery shopping and the time from the grocery store to home.

Let's Make a Meal

Simple meals can be healthy, but they don't have to include bland foods. Nutritious fare doesn't require expensive ingredients, and it doesn't require a ton of time to prepare and clean up after, either. To serve nutritious and delicious meals on a daily basis, it's important to get into a routine that works for you. Variety is important, and while you shouldn't eat the same foods every day, it's not necessary to try new recipes all the time, although there is nothing wrong with that approach.

Consider the recipes in this chapter as guidelines for good nutrition and great taste, but don't hesitate to make them your own. Personalize them by adding more or less herbs, spices, or salt, by substituting beans or tofu for chicken or beef, and by using whatever ingredients you have in the house, like asparagus for broccoli, and pasta instead of rice.

Detailed nutrition information is provided to help you account for calories, fat, saturated fat, cholesterol, carbohydrate, fiber, protein, and calcium. MyPlate doesn't focus on individual nutrients, so why provide the information? Because some people need to track certain nutrients to manage or prevent health conditions, including diabetes, heart disease, and osteoporosis.

You'll notice that the recipes yield different serving sizes. That's because households differ in size. If you need more food, double the recipe. Need less? Most recipes are divisible by half, and if not, put what you don't need in the freezer for future use.

We begin with dinner, typically the most daunting meal of the day because it requires the most planning.

Dinner: Plan to Succeed

Healthy dinners don't magically appear, as much as we would like them to. When you wait until late in the day to figure out what's for dinner, you'll surely scramble to put something nutritious, or not, on the table. Planning prevents the daily dinnertime dilemma.

Planning takes time, so it may seem like a chore, especially in the beginning. In the long run, planning for healthy meals and snacks saves time and money: there's no dashing to the store for dinner ingredients on a daily basis, and, in reducing your reliance on more expensive take-out and convenience foods, you'll conserve cash, and get a more nutritious diet in the bargain, too.

Get It and Forget It

Take time on the weekends to figure out what you need to have in the house for the week ahead. Then shop for the ingredients and cross that task off your to-do list.

☐ Cook Once, Eat Twice

You're already cooking, so make extra. Double up on your favorite chili, lasagna, or stew. Roast a whole chicken, serve it with vegetables and grains one night, and make chicken and cheese quesadillas the next.

These, and other kitchen staples, provide you with the raw materials to rustle up quick and healthy meals in minutes. Take this shopping list on your next trip to the supermarket, and add to it as needed to make meals and snacks for the week ahead, based on family favorites, and the recipes in this chapter.

- [ ] Canned tuna and canned salmon
- [ ] Eggs, preferably fortified eggs, such as Eggland's Best
- [ ] Fat-free and low-fat plain yogurt, including Greek yogurt, such as Chobani
- [ ] Frozen fish fillets, frozen shrimp
- [ ] Boneless, skinless chicken breasts
- [ ] Canned beans, such as garbanzo, black beans, and cannelloni
- [ ] Grated hard cheese, such as reduced-fat cheddar
- [ ] 95% lean ground beef
- [ ] Ground 100% turkey breast meat
- [ ] Low-fat cottage cheese, such as Lactaid brand (for those with lactose intolerance) and no-sodium added cottage cheese
- [ ] Fat-free and low-fat (1%) milk
- [ ] Whole-grain cereal
- [ ] Whole-grain breads
- [ ] Pasta, including whole wheat
- [ ] Rice, including brown rice
- [ ] Frozen fruit and fruit canned in its own juice
- [ ] Frozen vegetables and canned vegetables marked "no sodium added," "low sodium," or "reduced sodium"
- [ ] Balsamic vinegar
- [ ] Olive oil and canola oil
- [ ] Marinara sauce
- [ ] Dried fruit, such as cranberries, cherries, and California raisins
- [ ] Nuts, including pistachios, almonds, walnuts, cashews, and peanuts
- [ ] Peanut butter, almond butter, or sunflower seed butter

Plan B

The evening meal can catch even the most organized person off-guard. Here's what to serve when your plans for a home cooked dinner go down in flames and you're rushing to put a healthy meal on the table.

- Rotisserie chicken; salad of pre-washed greens, cherry tomatoes, and olives; quick-cooking grain, such as whole-wheat couscous
- Thin-crust frozen whole-grain pizza, fruit salad, milk (Keep a thin crust whole-grain frozen pizza on hand to prevent the urge to order a take-out deep dish pie with everything on it.)
- Breakfast for dinner ("brinner"): French toast made with whole-grain bread, fruit, milk; scrambled eggs, whole-grain toast, vegetables, milk; whole-grain frozen waffles topped with low-fat vanilla yogurt and fruit, such as sliced strawberries, milk
- Frozen spinach and cheese pie (cook at home), rice (cook while spinach pie is in the oven), fruit, milk
- Burgers made with 100% ground turkey breast or 95% lean ground beef, on whole-wheat buns; salad with pre-washed greens, mandarin oranges, sliced almonds, milk
- Pasta and prepared marinara sauce combined with leftover chopped roasted or grilled chicken or canned, drained garbanzo beans added to it; fruit, milk

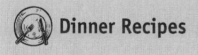 **Dinner Recipes**

Crispy Pistachio Chicken
Makes 4 servings.

You'll love the crunch the pistachios provide, as well as the heart-healthy fat.

3 tablespoons canola oil
2 tablespoons grated fresh ginger root
2 tablespoons lemon juice
1 tablespoon honey

4 cloves garlic, peeled and minced
1 teaspoon paprika
1 pound boneless, skinless chicken breasts
¾ cup unsalted, shelled California pistachios, chopped finely or ground
½ cup plain breadcrumbs
1 large egg, beaten

Preheat oven to 400°F.

In a small bowl, combine canola oil, ginger, lemon juice, honey, garlic, and paprika. Toss with chicken, cover, and marinate in refrigerator for at least one hour. In small shallow bowl, mix pistachios and breadcrumbs. Pour egg into small shallow bowl. Dip each piece of marinated chicken first into the egg, then in pistachio mixture, pressing the nuts onto the chicken, if necessary. Bake for 25 minutes or until done.

Per serving: 449 calories; 24 grams carbohydrate; 3 grams fiber; 24 grams fat; 5 grams saturated fat; 35 grams protein; 192 milligrams sodium; 118 milligrams cholesterol; 70 milligrams calcium.

• •

Slow Cooker Middle Eastern Stew
Makes 6 servings.

The herbs and spices in this delicious dish add flavor and keep the sodium count low. Serve with whole-wheat couscous and a green salad for a complete meal.

¼ cup olive oil
8 boneless, skinless chicken thighs, cut into 1-inch cubes
1 eggplant, peeled, cut into 2-inch cubes
3 onions, peeled and thinly sliced
4 carrots, peeled and thinly sliced
4 cloves garlic, peeled and minced
½ cup dried apricots, chopped
2 cups low-sodium chicken broth
2 tablespoons tomato paste
2 tablespoons lemon juice
2 tablespoons all-purpose flour
1½ teaspoons ground cumin
1½ teaspoons ground ginger
1½ teaspoons ground cinnamon
1 cup water

In a heavy skillet, heat half the olive oil over medium-high heat. Add half the chicken to pan and brown on all sides. Do not cook all the way through. Repeat with the remaining oil and chicken. Place browned chicken in the bottom of a slow cooker. Place eggplant, onions, carrots, garlic, and apricots over the chicken.

In a medium bowl, whisk together the chicken broth, tomato paste, lemon juice, flour, cumin, ginger, cinnamon, and water until blended thoroughly. Pour the mixture into the slow cooker. Cook on high for about 5 hours.

Per serving: 331 calories; 21 grams carbohydrate; 5 grams fiber; 21 grams fat; 5 grams saturated fat; 16 grams protein; 275 milligrams sodium; 64 milligrams cholesterol; 50 milligrams calcium.

• •

Chicken Piccata

Makes 4 servings.

This tasty dish pairs well with angel hair pasta and roasted asparagus.

1 pound boneless, skinless chicken breasts
¼ teaspoon fresh ground black pepper
½ cup all-purpose flour
4 tablespoons trans-fat free tub margarine
2 tablespoons olive oil
⅓ cup lemon juice
½ cup low-sodium chicken broth
2 tablespoons brined capers, rinsed
⅓ cup fresh parsley, chopped (optional)

Season chicken with the pepper. Coat each piece of chicken with flour and shake off the excess. In a large skillet, over medium heat, melt 2 tablespoons of margarine in the pan. Add 1 tablespoon olive oil and stir. Brown chicken, about 3 minutes on each side. Remove chicken from the pan and set aside. Melt the remaining margarine, add oil and repeat until all of the chicken is browned.

Add the lemon juice, chicken broth, and capers to the pan. Bring the mixture to a boil, scraping down brown bits from the pan for extra flavor. Return the chicken to the pan and simmer for 5 minutes or until done. Place chicken on a platter. Pour sauce over chicken; garnish with parsley.

Per serving: 390 calories; 13 grams carbohydrate; 1 gram fiber;

25 grams fat; 5 grams saturated fat; 28 grams protein; 299 milligrams sodium; 65 milligrams cholesterol; 20 milligrams calcium.

• •

Coconut Chicken Tenders
Makes 4 servings.

The sweetness of the coconut balances the seasoned breadcrumbs and provides a satisfying crunch to this fun finger food.

½ cup all-purpose flour
½ cup shredded coconut
½ cup seasoned Panko breadcrumbs
1 large egg
1 cup low-fat (1%) milk
1 pound boneless skinless chicken breast, cut into 1-inch strips
2 tablespoons canola oil

Place flour in one-quart resealable plastic food storage bag. In a separate food storage bag, combine the coconut and breadcrumbs, seal bag and shake to mix well. In a medium shallow bowl, combine the egg and milk. Mix well. Working in batches, add the chicken to the flour bag and coat well, then dip each piece in the egg mixture and place in the bag with the coconut and breadcrumbs and shake to coat chicken.

Heat a 12-inch skillet over medium-high heat. Add 1 tablespoon oil to pan and heat. Add chicken to pan and cook five minutes, flip and cook for 2 to 3 minutes on the other side. Repeat with remaining oil and chicken.

Serve with *Apricot Dijon Mustard Spread*, page 133, if desired.

Per serving (without the apricot spread): 401 calories; 31 grams carbohydrate; 2 grams fiber; 15 grams fat; 6 grams saturated fat; 34 grams protein; 412 milligrams sodium; 121 milligrams cholesterol; 120 milligrams calcium.

• •

Steak Tacos with Salsamole
Makes 6 tacos.

These steak tacos are simple and satisfying, and pair well with fruit salad.

½ teaspoon salt
pinch of each: fresh ground black pepper, crushed red pepper, dried thyme, dried rosemary, onion powder

1½ pounds top sirloin steak, trimmed
8 (8-inch) tortillas

Salsamole (see recipe on page 157)

Heat the grill, or coat a 12-inch skillet with cooking spray and heat over medium-high heat.

In a small bowl, combine the salt with the pepper, red pepper, thyme, rosemary, and onion powder. Rub the steaks with the salt mixture. Grill or broil the steaks for 5 minutes on each side, turning once. Remove from the heat and let rest. Cut into thin slices and keep warm.

To make tacos, spread salsamole on each tortilla, top with sliced steak and roll up or fold into quarters to eat.

Per serving (1 taco): 357 calories; 31 grams carbohydrate; 3 grams fiber; 12 grams fat; 3 grams saturated fat; 31 grams protein; 788 milligrams sodium; 40 milligrams cholesterol; 140 milligrams calcium.

● ●

Chocolate Chili
Makes 6 servings.

Unsweetened cocoa powder pumps up the flavor and the flavonoids – plant compounds that protect your cells—in this recipe. Serve with crusty whole-grain rolls and a green salad.

1 pound ground sirloin or ground 100% turkey breast
2 tablespoons olive or canola oil
4 cloves garlic, peeled and diced
1 medium onion, peeled and chopped
1 green or red bell pepper, seeded and chopped
1 (16-ounce) can reduced-sodium black beans, drained and rinsed
1 (16-ounce) can reduced-sodium red kidney beans, drained and rinsed
1 (28-ounce) no-salt-added diced tomatoes, undrained
½ teaspoon ground cumin
1 tablespoon unsweetened cocoa (optional)

Place a 6-quart saucepan over medium-high heat. Add the meat. Brown the meat, breaking it up into very small pieces as it cooks. Drain. Remove the meat from the pan and reserve. Season with salt and ground black pepper, if desired. Return the pan to the stove. Add the oil to pan and heat over medium heat. Add the garlic, onion, and pepper and cook until soft, about 5 minutes. Add the meat back to pan, and stir in the beans, tomatoes, cumin, and cocoa. Heat to boiling, then reduce heat and simmer for 10 to 15 minutes.

Per serving: 286 calories; 29 grams carbohydrate; 9 grams fiber; 2 grams fat; 2 grams saturated fat; 25 grams protein; 331 milligrams sodium; 46 milligrams cholesterol; 80 milligrams calcium.

• •

Almost Lasagna
Makes 6 servings.

This recipe has all the elements of lasagna without the fuss. Substitute tofu or 100% ground turkey breast for a change.

1 pound long fusilli pasta or linguine
1 pound 95% lean ground beef
2 tablespoons extra virgin olive oil
1 small carrot, grated or finely chopped
1 small onion, grated or finely chopped
2 cloves garlic, grated or finely chopped
1 cup low-sodium beef broth
1 (28-ounce) can no-salt-added crushed tomatoes
fresh basil leaves, torn
½ cup low-fat ricotta cheese
⅓ cup chopped flat-leaf parsley, or 2 teaspoons dried parsley
2 tablespoons trans-fat free margarine

Bring a large pot of water to a boil, add the pasta, and cook until al dente. Drain.

Meanwhile, heat a large skillet over medium heat. Add the beef, crumbling it into bits, and cook until lightly browned, about 3 to 4 minutes. Remove the skillet from the heat and drain the meat, then transfer meat to a medium bowl and reserve. Return the skillet to the stove, add the olive oil, and heat over medium heat. Add the carrot, onion, and garlic and cook until the vegetables are softened, about 5 minutes. Season with salt and fresh ground black pepper, if desired. Add the meat back to the pan. Stir in the broth, tomatoes, and basil; simmer for five minutes.

In a small bowl, stir together the ricotta cheese and parsley. Toss the pasta with the margarine and return to skillet. Mix with meat sauce. To serve, scoop equal amounts of the ricotta into shallow bowls, and top with the pasta and sauce.

Per serving: 483 calories; 64 grams carbohydrate; 4 grams fiber; 11 grams fat; 4 grams saturated fat; 30 grams protein; 108 milligrams sodium; 108 milligrams cholesterol; 120 milligrams calcium.

● ●

Pork, Asparagus, and Cashew Stir Fry
Makes 6 servings.

Pork tenderloin is as lean and low in calories as boneless, skinless chicken breast. Cashews provide flavor, crunch, and heart-healthy fats.

1 bunch of asparagus, trimmed, and cut into 1-inch pieces
1 cup low-sodium chicken broth
¼ cup rice wine vinegar
1 tablespoon sugar
¼ cup low-sodium soy sauce
3 tablespoons cornstarch, divided
1 pound pork tenderloin, trimmed
3 tablespoons canola oil, divided
6 cloves garlic, peeled and minced
1 tablespoon fresh grated ginger
1 cup unsalted cashews, chopped

Cook asparagus until crisp-tender. Do not overcook.

In a medium bowl, whisk the chicken broth, vinegar, sugar, and 1 tablespoon cornstarch until no lumps remain. Set aside.

Cut pork into ½-inch medallions, then cut each medallion into ½-inch-thick strips. Add pork to a large bowl and toss with 1 tablespoon oil. Add remaining 2 tablespoons cornstarch to pork mixture and toss to coat the meat.

In a 12-inch skillet, heat 1 tablespoon oil over medium-high heat. Cook half the pork, about 3 to 5 minutes. Remove from skillet and set aside, covered, on a plate. Repeat with remaining oil and pork. Remove pork from pan.

Add asparagus to pan, along with garlic and ginger. Cook for 30 seconds. Stir broth mixture before adding to skillet. Cook until thickened, about 2 minutes. Add pork and cashews to pan and cook until heated through, about 1 to 2 minutes.

Per serving: 308 calories; 14 grams carbohydrate; 2 grams fiber; 19 grams fat; 3 grams saturated fat; 22 grams protein; 410 milligrams sodium; 49 milligrams cholesterol; 30 milligrams calcium.

Baked Salmon with Pineapple Salsa

Makes 4 servings.

Salmon harbors omega-3 fats. Keep frozen fillets on hand for a quick weeknight meal.

1 pound skinless salmon fillets, 1-inch thick
2 teaspoons olive oil
3 tablespoons salt-free garlic and herb blend
½ cup diced green peppers
½ cup diced red peppers
1 cup canned, drained crushed pineapple
½ teaspoon ground ginger

Preheat oven to 425°F.

Arrange salmon fillets on a baking sheet lined with aluminum foil. Sprinkle fillets with equal amounts of olive oil and garlic and herb blend. Bake fish for about 10 - 15 minutes or until fish flakes easily. Meanwhile, in a medium microwavable bowl, combine green and red peppers, pineapple, and ginger. Mix well. Heat salsa for 45 seconds on high. Top cooked salmon with pineapple salsa.

Per serving: 290 calories; 9 grams carbohydrate; 1 gram fiber; 17 grams fat; 4 grams saturated fat; 23 grams protein; 68 milligrams sodium; 62 milligrams cholesterol; 20 milligrams calcium.

Tilapia Tacos

Makes 8 tacos.

Have you tried tilapia? It's mild in taste, affordable, and widely available. You may prefer it to stronger-tasting seafood.

1 pound tilapa
¼ teaspoon ground red pepper
¼ teaspoon garlic powder
3 tablespoons olive oil
8 (8-inch) tortillas
1 medium tomato, chopped
1 large avocado, peeled and sliced
Shredded lettuce
6 tablespoons fat-free Ranch dressing

Season the tilapia with red pepper and garlic powder. Heat olive oil in a 12-inch nonstick skillet over medium heat. Add the fish and sauté until fish is opaque. Break cooked fish into pieces with a fork.

Fill 8 tortillas with fish and equal amounts of chopped tomato, avocado, and shredded lettuce, and 3 teaspoons Ranch dressing. Roll up to eat.

Per serving (2 tacos): 392 calories; 42 grams carbohydrate; 3 grams fiber; 17 grams fat; 4 grams saturated fat; 19 grams protein; 469 milligrams sodium; 29 milligrams cholesterol; 150 milligrams calcium.

•••

Roasted Shrimp and Orzo Salad

Makes 6 servings.

Roasting shrimp enhances its flavor.

1 pound raw shrimp, peeled and deveined
1½ teaspoons olive oil
1 cup orzo, uncooked
3 tablespoons olive oil
½ teaspoon salt
3 tablespoons lemon juice
¼ teaspoon fresh ground black pepper
1 (9-ounce) package frozen plain artichokes, thawed
½ cup (2 ounces) feta cheese, crumbled
1 cup no-salt added, low-fat cottage cheese
2 cups grape or cherry tomatoes, cut in half
1 tablespoon chopped fresh dill or 1 teaspoon dried dill

Preheat oven to 400°F.

Place shrimp in a single layer on a rimmed baking sheet and drizzle with 1½ teaspoons olive oil. Sprinkle with fresh ground black pepper, if desired. Roast for 5 minutes.

Cook orzo according to package directions. Drain and rinse with cold water. Add to a large serving bowl. Add three tablespoons olive oil, salt, lemon juice, and pepper and toss to coat orzo. Add artichokes, feta cheese, cottage cheese, tomatoes, and roasted shrimp. Garnish with dill and serve or refrigerate.

Per serving: 299 calories; 12 grams carbohydrate; 3 grams fiber; 13 grams fat; 4 grams saturated fat; 25 grams protein; 472 milligrams sodium; 126 milligrams cholesterol; 140 milligrams calcium.

Egg and Artichoke Pie
Makes 6 servings.

Eggs are versatile, convenient, and provide relatively more nutrition for the calories and for your food dollar. This is a good-for-you pie that tastes great as a leftover.

1 (10-inch) whole-wheat tortilla
2 tablespoons trans-fat free tub margarine
1 small onion, peeled and chopped
4 cloves garlic, peeled and minced
1 (9-ounce) package frozen plain artichoke hearts, thawed
¼ cup chopped fresh parsley or 2 teaspoons dried parsley
½ teaspoon fresh ground black pepper
2 large eggs
1 cup low-fat (1%) milk
1 cup all-purpose flour
1 teaspoon baking powder
½ teaspoon salt
1 cup shredded reduced-fat cheddar cheese

Preheat the oven to 425°F. Grease a 9-inch pie plate. Press the tortilla into the pie plate.

In a medium skillet, heat the margarine over medium heat. Add the onions and garlic and sauté until the onions are translucent. Remove from heat.

In a medium bowl, toss the artichokes with the parsley and pepper. In another medium bowl, whisk together the eggs, milk, flour, baking powder, and salt.

Sprinkle half the cheese in the pie pan. Add the artichoke mixture. Slowly pour the egg mixture into the pie plate. Sprinkle with remaining cheese.

Bake for 20 minutes or until a knife inserted in the center comes out clean. Cool on a wire rack for 5 minutes before serving.

Per serving: 182 calories; 20 grams carbohydrate; 4 grams fiber; 7 grams fat; 3 grams saturated fat; 11 grams protein; 788 milligrams sodium; 76 milligrams cholesterol; 200 milligrams calcium.

Bean 'N Cheese Enchiladas
Makes 4 servings.

A serving has as much calcium as a glass of milk, and more than three times the protein. Substitute leftover beans for canned beans.

1½ cups no-salt-added low-fat cottage cheese
1 cup shredded reduced fat cheddar cheese, divided
1 cup canned black beans, rinsed and drained
¾ teaspoon dried oregano
½ cup fresh tomato salsa
8 (8-inch) flour tortillas

Preheat oven to 375° F.

Coat a 12- x 8-inch baking dish with cooking spray.

Blend cottage cheese in food processor or blender until smooth. Transfer to a large mixing bowl. Stir in ½ cup cheddar cheese, beans, and oregano. Place about ⅓ cup cheese mixture in center of each tortilla, and roll up. Place each tortilla in baking dish with the seam side facing down. Top tortillas with salsa, then with the remaining cheese. Bake for 20 to 25 minutes or until thoroughly heated.

Per serving: 462 calories; 62 grams carbohydrate; 7 grams fiber; 10 grams fat; 4 grams saturated fat; 29 grams protein; 1066 milligrams sodium; 9 milligrams cholesterol; 310 milligrams calcium.

Pasta with Sundried Tomatoes, Spinach, and Garbanzo Beans
Makes 4 servings.

Here's a quick vegetarian dish that will win raves from your family. Top with crumbled feta cheese for a Mediterranean flair.

8 ounces whole-wheat ziti pasta, uncooked
8 pieces sundried tomatoes, chopped into ¼-inch pieces
¼ cup hot or boiling water
2 tablespoons olive oil
10 ounces fresh baby spinach (about 10 cups packed leaves)
1 (15.5-ounce) can cannellini beans (white kidney beans), drained and rinsed

Cook pasta according to package directions. Drain and keep warm.

Meanwhile, in a small bowl, soak tomatoes in ¼ cup hot or boiling water for about 5 minutes. Do not discard fluid.

In a 12-inch skillet, heat olive oil over medium heat. Add half the spinach and cook until just wilted. Remove from pan and reserve. Repeat with remaining spinach. Add first batch of spinach back to the pan. Add tomatoes and their soaking liquid and the beans. Toss to combine well. Add warm pasta to the pan and toss to coat. Serve.

Per serving: 375 calories; 64 grams carbohydrate; 11 grams fiber; 8 grams fat; 1 gram saturated fat; 17 grams protein; 307 milligrams sodium; 0 milligrams cholesterol; 160 milligrams calcium.

• •

Haddock In a Packet
Makes 4 servings.

So simple, yet so delicious!

1½ pounds haddock, skin removed
½ cup seasoned breadcrumbs
3 tablespoons olive oil
3 cups cherry tomatoes, cut in half
2 teaspoons dried parsley

Preheat oven to 400°F.

Line 9-x 13-inch roasting pan with aluminum foil, leaving enough to form a packet, about 12-inches hanging over each side of the pan, lengthwise. Place the fish in the pan.

Sprinkle the fish with the breadcrumbs. Drizzle with olive oil; top with tomatoes and parsley.

Form a packet with the aluminum foil. Bake for 20 to 25 minutes, or until fish flakes easily with a fork.

Per serving: 313 calories; 15 grams carbohydrate; 2 grams fiber; 12 grams fat; 2 grams saturated fat; 35 grams protein; 384 milligrams sodium; 96 milligrams cholesterol; 90 milligrams calcium.

Pizza, please!

Americans love pizza. Unfortunately, pizza is a major contributor of saturated fat in our diets. Pizza is simple, satisfying, and convenient, and can be rich in whole grains, calcium, fiber, and many other nutrients. The problem is, stuffed crusts, extra cheese, and fatty meat toppings turn pizza into a dietary disaster. That's why pizza gets its own section in this chapter.

It's possible to build healthier pies at home instead of always ordering take-out and relying on frozen pizza. With pizza, there are dozens of "out-of-the box" combinations that taste great, and are better for you. All you need is your imagination to come up with pies that stretch the boundaries of traditional tomato and cheese pizza. Or, if you're not feeling adventurous, stick with simple pie that you love, only make it healthier!

First, the foundation. Choose whole-grain crusts to help meet the daily suggested minimum of three servings.

• Store-bought or homemade pizza dough
• Store-bought frozen bread dough, thawed
• Pre-cooked thin pizza crust
• English muffin
• Bagel
• Deli flats thin bread or sandwich thins
• Tortilla or other sandwich wrap
• Pita bread
• Naan

Get saucy. Stick with tomato sauce, try any one of the following options, or go sauce-free.
• Equal amounts of prepared pesto sauce and Greek yogurt
• Reduced-fat cream cheese (spread on warm, cooked crust, then add toppings)
• Hummus (spread on warm, cooked crust, then add toppings)

Choose your cheese. Cheese packs protein and calcium, but it's also mostly to blame for pizza's high calorie and sodium counts as well as total and saturated fat content. To curb calories and fat, limit cheese; use less of the lower-fat cheese varieties for even further reductions. Top each large pie with about eight ounces of cheese, and no more than two ounces for a single-serving pizza.

- Part-skim mozzarella cheese
- 50% reduced-fat cheddar cheese
- Reduced-fat feta cheese
- Blue cheese
- Fontina cheese

Pick your protein. Save calories and sodium by giving up the fatty meat toppings for higher-protein, lower-fat choices.

- Cooked, shredded chicken
- Crumbled apple chicken sausage
- Reduced-sodium ham, Canadian bacon, or proscuitto
- Cooked, flaked salmon
- Cooked, chopped clams
- Cooked shrimp

Top it off. Fruits and veggies add flavor and fiber for relatively few calories.

- Veggie suggestions: cooked asparagus, artichokes, eggplant, roasted red peppers, raw or cooked broccoli, onions, olives, raw baby spinach or arugula, artichokes, cooked zucchini, sliced tomatoes, thinly-sliced fennel
- Pineapple chunks, sliced pears, sliced apples, mandarin oranges

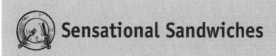

Sensational Sandwiches

Sandwiches are fine fare for any meal of the day. There's no need to stress about preparing a time-consuming entrée when you have delicious ingredients on hand to nestle between two slices of bread, stuffed into a bread pocket or bun, or to display on flatbread.

Egg and Mushroom Pita Pocket

Makes 1 serving.

Make this in minutes for breakfast, lunch, or dinner.

1 teaspoon olive oil
1 large egg, beaten
½ cup white button mushrooms, sliced
½ (7-inch) pita pocket
¼ cup shredded reduced-fat cheddar cheese

Coat a small skillet with nonstick cooking spray. Add oil over medium heat. Add egg and mushrooms and scramble. To assemble, place cooked egg/mushroom mixture in pita pocket. Top with cheese.

Per serving: 261 calories; 20 grams carbohydrate; 3 grams fiber; 13 grams fat; 4 grams saturated fat; 19 grams protein; 444 milligrams sodium; 218 milligrams cholesterol; 170 milligrams calcium.

• •

Easy Pulled Pork Sandwiches

Makes 6 servings.

Skip the bread and serve this no-fuss pulled pork over white rice.

1¾ pounds pork tenderloin, trimmed
1 teaspoon chili powder
1 teaspoon paprika
½ teaspoon fresh ground black pepper
2 tablespoons canola oil
¼ cup low-sodium chicken broth
½ cup prepared barbecue sauce
3 tablespoons cider vinegar

6 whole-wheat English muffins, toasted or 6 (2-ounce) whole-grain sandwich buns

Slice the pork tenderloin into 1-inch thick medallions and place in medium bowl. In a small bowl, combine the chili powder, paprika, and pepper. Add the spice mixture to the meat and toss to coat thoroughly.

Heat 1 tablespoon oil in a 12-inch skillet over medium-high heat. Working in batches, add the pork, and cook until browned, about 5 minutes each side. Transfer cooked meat to a plate and cover. Add remaining oil to pan and cook remaining pork.

Using 2 forks, shred meat into bite-size pieces.

To make sauce, add the broth, barbecue sauce, and vinegar to skillet. Simmer over medium-low heat until sauce has thickened, scraping up any browned bits in the pan, about 3 minutes. Add pork back to skillet and cook for about 3 minutes or until heated through.

To serve, divide pork equally among the English muffins or buns.

Per serving (with English muffin): 355 calories; 31 grams carbohydrate; 4 grams fiber; 9 grams fat; 2 grams saturated fat; 35 grams protein; 570 milligrams sodium; 85 milligrams cholesterol; 70 milligrams calcium.

● ●

Crab and Avocado Flatbread Sandwich
Makes 2 servings.

Canned crab is a convenient low-fat protein source that provides much-needed omega-3 fats. It pairs well with creamy avocado.

1 tablespoon low-fat mayonnaise
¼ teaspoon fresh ground black pepper
1 (6-ounce) can crab meat, drained
2 pieces roasted jarred red pepper, drained and chopped
1 piece naan bread (about 4 ounces) or other thin flat-bread
½ large fresh avocado, peeled and sliced

In a small bowl, combine mayonnaise and pepper.

In another small bowl, mix crab meat and red pepper.

Toast the bread, then spread with mayonnaise mixture. Top with crabmeat mixture and sliced avocado. Divide flatbread in two.

Per serving: 348 calories; 41 grams carbohydrate; 6 grams fiber; 12 grams fat; 0 grams saturated fat; 20 grams protein; 632 milligrams sodium; 59 milligrams cholesterol; 120 milligrams calcium.

• •

Salmon Salad
Makes 4 servings.

Salmon salad makes it simple to include the 8 ounces or more of seafood in your diet suggested in the 2010 Dietary Guidelines for Americans. Serve salmon over a bed of fresh spinach or romaine lettuce for a change of pace.

12 ounces of boneless, skinless salmon from a can or pouch, or other cooked salmon
½ cup Panko breadcrumbs
½ cup minced red onion
2 tablespoons lemon juice
1 tablespoon low-fat mayonnaise
¼ teaspoon freshly ground pepper
8 slices pumpernickel bread
8 large tomato slices
4 large romaine lettuce leaves

In a medium bowl, combine salmon, breadcrumbs, onion, lemon juice, mayonnaise, and pepper.

Place equal amounts of salmon salad on 4 slices of bread; top with 2 slices tomato and romaine leaves. Top with remaining bread slices.

Per serving (one sandwich): 347 calories; 40 grams carbohydrate; 5 grams fiber; 8 grams fat; 1 gram saturated fat; 30 grams protein; 804 milligrams sodium; 59 milligrams cholesterol; 90 milligrams calcium.

Per serving (¼ recipe without bread): 206 calories; 12 grams carbohydrate; 1 gram fiber; 6 grams fat; 1 gram saturated fat; 25 grams protein; 425 milligrams sodium; 59 milligrams cholesterol; 50 milligrams calcium.

• •

Chicken, Apple, and Cheese Panini
Makes 4 sandwiches.

Apricot Dijon Mustard Spread
½ cup apricot preserves
1 teaspoon Dijon mustard

8 ounces sliced cooked, boneless, skinless chicken breast
4 ounces reduced-fat sharp cheddar cheese, or other hard cheese
½ apple or pear, with skin, sliced into ⅛-inch slices
8 slices country bread or ciabatta
4 teaspoons trans-fat free tub margarine

To make spread: In a small bowl, combine apricot preserves and mustard.

Place equal amounts of the apricot spread on one side of the four pieces of bread. Layer equal amounts of the chicken, cheese, and fruit on top. Top with the remaining bread.

Heat a 12-inch nonstick skillet over medium heat. Coat skillet with cooking spray. Add two teaspoons of margarine to the pan. Cook two of the sandwiches until golden and crisp, about 3 to 4 minutes each side. Repeat for remaining sandwiches. Or, preheat a panini press and cook sandwiches according to manufacturer's instructions.

Per serving: 408 calories; 54 grams carbohydrate; 2 grams fiber; 9 grams fat; 4 grams saturated fat; 29 grams protein; 623 milligrams sodium; 53 milligrams cholesterol; 170 milligrams calcium.

• •

Eggs Florentine Wrap
Makes 1 sandwich.

Keep the cooking to a minimum and maximize nutrition with this wrap sandwich.

1 egg
1 tablespoon feta cheese
1 tablespoon trans-fat free tub margarine
¼ medium onion, diced
1 cup fresh baby spinach, packed, roughly chopped
1 (7- to 8-inch) whole-wheat tortilla or sandwich wrap
fresh ground black pepper, to taste

In a medium bowl, beat egg. Add feta cheese and set aside.

Heat a large skillet over medium heat. Add half the margarine. Add onions and cook until translucent. Add spinach to the pan and cook until just wilted, about one minute. Place onion and spinach mixture in a small bowl and set aside. Add remaining margarine to skillet, lower heat to medium-low, and add the egg mixture. Scramble egg mixture until cooked. Add spinach and onion mixture back to pan and mix with eggs. Place this mixture in the center of the tortilla. Roll up to eat.

Per serving: 263 calories; 18 grams carbohydrate; 3 grams fiber; 17 grams fat; 6 grams saturated fat; 12 grams protein; 439 milligrams sodium; 219 milligrams cholesterol; 120 milligrams calcium.

● ●

Tuna Patties on Whole-Wheat English Muffins
Makes 4 sandwiches.

Use fresh tuna steak instead of canned tuna, if you like. Rely on canned light tuna, or a mixture of canned and light tuna if you're a woman in your childbearing years.

2 (6-ounce) cans solid white tuna, drained, or ½ cup flaked, cooked tuna
½ cup Panko breadcrumbs
2 large eggs
½ cup chopped red onion
½ cup chopped celery
2 teaspoons prepared horseradish
½ teaspoon fresh ground black pepper
1 tablespoon low-fat mayonnaise
2 tablespoons olive oil
4 whole-wheat English muffins, toasted, *or*
    2-ounce whole-grain sandwich buns

Preheat the oven to 350°F.

In a large bowl, combine the first 8 ingredients (tuna through mayonnaise). Form the mixture into four patties. Heat oil in a 12-inch nonstick skillet over medium heat. Cook the patties until golden brown on one side. Flip and cook for another five minutes. Remove from pan and place on baking sheet coated with cooking spray. Bake for 5 minutes.

Per serving: 375 calories; 29 grams carbohydrate; 4 grams fiber; 15 grams fat; 3 grams saturated fat; 31 grams protein; 403 milligrams sodium; 143 milligrams cholesterol; 100 milligrams calcium.

Turkey Burgers

Makes 6 burgers (or 18 meatballs*).

This versatile recipe turns out delicious burgers and meatballs. Double the recipe, serving burgers at one meal, and meatballs at a later meal. (Freeze meatballs until ready to use.)

½ cup low-fat cottage cheese**
1 tablespoon low-fat (1%) milk
1 pound ground 100% turkey breast
1 large egg
½ cup seasoned breadcrumbs
2 teaspoons dried basil or ¼ cup chopped fresh basil
½ teaspoon fresh ground black pepper
2 tablespoons canola oil
4 (2-ounce) whole-wheat sandwich buns

Place cottage cheese and milk in blender or food processor and blend until smooth, about 1 minute.

In a large bowl, combine the cottage cheese mixture with the remaining ingredients, except for the canola oil and buns, and mix well. Form mixture into 6 burgers.

Heat a 12-inch nonstick skillet over medium-high heat. (Or grill burgers.) Add canola oil. Cook burgers for about 5 to 7 minutes on each side, or until a meat thermometer inserted in the middle of the burger registers 165°F. Serve on sandwich buns.

* *To make meatballs, divide meat mixture into 18 balls. Brown in a skillet in canola oil over medium-high heat. Bake in preheated 375°F oven for 12 to15 minutes.*
** *You can substitute low-fat ricotta cheese for cottage cheese. Do not process with milk in the blender or food processor. Add ricotta cheese directly to meat mixture.*

Per serving: 340 calories; 36 grams carbohydrate; 5 grams fiber; 10 grams fat; 2 grams saturated fat; 27 grams protein; 579 milligrams sodium; 81 milligrams cholesterol; 100 milligrams calcium.

Per serving (3 meatballs): 191 calories; 7 grams carbohydrate; 0 grams fiber; 7 grams fat; 2 grams saturated fat; 22 grams protein; 311 milligrams sodium; 81 milligrams cholesterol; 40 milligrams calcium.

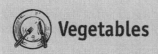 **Vegetables**

Do you eat enough vegetables? Probably not. Maybe you think they're a pain to prepare, or you're bored with your usual choices. The following recipes offer a new perspective on old favorites, and provide a twist or two to pique your interest in a variety of produce.

Smashed Yukon Gold Potatoes with Garlic and Chives
Makes 6 servings.

Yukon Gold potatoes are creamier than most, so you can use less fat when making mashed potatoes.

1¼ pounds Yukon Gold potatoes, cut into 1-inch pieces
3 cloves garlic, peeled
¼ cup low-sodium vegetable broth, warmed
½ cup low-fat sour cream
2 tablespoons trans-fat free tub margarine
3 tablespoons chopped fresh chives
¼ teaspoon fresh ground black pepper

Bring water to boil in large saucepan. Add potatoes and garlic. Cook until potatoes are tender, about 15 minutes. When done, drain and return to pan. Add broth, sour cream, margarine, chives, and pepper; mash.

Per serving: 129 calories; 18 grams carbohydrate; 2 grams fiber; 2 grams fat; 0 grams saturated fat; 3 grams protein; 47 milligrams sodium; 8 milligrams cholesterol; 30 milligrams calcium.

• •

Portabello Mushroom Parmesan
Makes 4 servings.

These mushrooms double as a side dish and an entrée.

4 large Portabello mushrooms, washed with stems removed
2 tablespoons olive oil
1 cup drained, canned no-salt-added chopped tomatoes
½ teaspoon dried basil
¼ teaspoon crushed red peppers flakes
1 cup (4 ounces) shredded part-skim mozzarella cheese

Preheat oven to 400°F.

In a 12-inch skillet, heat oil over medium-high heat. Add mushrooms to pan and cook for about 3 to 4 minutes each side.

Spread ½ cup of the tomatoes on the bottom of medium baking dish. Place mushrooms, gill sides up in dish. Sprinkle with basil, red pepper flakes, and remaining tomatoes. Top each mushroom with equal amounts of cheese. Bake for 5 to 10 minutes, or until the cheese begins to brown.

Per serving: 177 calories; 8 grams carbohydrate; 2 grams fiber; 13 grams fat; 5 grams saturated fat; 10 grams protein; 160 milligrams sodium; 15 milligrams cholesterol; 230 milligrams calcium.

• •

Minestrone in Minutes
Makes 6 servings.

Soup is an easy way to work in much-needed vegetables.

2 teaspoons olive oil
1 medium onion, peeled and chopped
3 cloves garlic, peeled and minced
3 cups low-sodium vegetable broth
1 (28-ounce) can no-salt-added diced tomatoes, undrained
1 (15-ounce) can white (cannellini or navy) beans, rinsed and drained
1 teaspoon dried thyme
1 teaspoon dried sage
¾ cup small macaroni, uncooked
3 cups frozen mixed vegetables, such as broccoli, cauliflower, and carrots
½ teaspoon salt
⅛ teaspoon fresh ground black pepper

Add oil to a small skillet over medium heat. Add onion and garlic and sauté until onion is translucent.

In a large saucepan, combine broth, tomatoes, beans, thyme, and sage. Bring to a simmer and add pasta, frozen vegetables, salt, and pepper. Cook for 6 minutes. Let soup sit for five minutes or more to allow the macaroni to finish cooking.

Per serving: 250 calories; 45 grams carbohydrate; 9 grams fiber; 3 grams fat; 1 gram saturated fat; 13 grams protein; 474 milligrams sodium; 0 milligrams cholesterol; 130 milligrams calcium.

Cream of Squash Soup

Makes 8 servings.

So creamy and delicious, you may forget you're eating your veggies! This also doubles as a delicious side dish, too.

2 tablespoons canola oil
1 large onion, peeled and chopped
1 teaspoon ground ginger
1 teaspoon ground cumin
½ teaspoon salt
1 cup low-sodium chicken or vegetable broth
6 cups cooked butternut squash (leftovers or frozen plain squash, thawed)
1 cup cooked sweet potato
2½ cups (2%) reduced-fat milk or fat-free half and half

In a large saucepan, heat oil over medium heat. Add onion and cook until translucent. Add ginger, cumin, salt, and broth. Stir until ingredients are well combined. Add squash and sweet potato. Stir thoroughly. Remove from heat and cool. Transfer squash mixture in batches to a food processor or blender and puree each batch until smooth, about 3 to 5 minutes. Return pureed mixture to saucepan. Add milk or half and half and heat gently until warm. Serve immediately.

Note: To make as a side dish, omit the milk or half and half.

Per serving (Made with 2% reduced-fat milk): 176 calories; 30 grams carbohydrate; 1 gram fiber; 5 grams fat; 1 gram saturated fat; 5 grams protein; 203 milligrams sodium; 6 milligrams cholesterol; 180 milligrams calcium.

Ramen Noodle Salad

Makes 8 servings.

Cabbage is the basis of this crunchy and refreshing dish.

Dressing:
2 tablespoons canola oil
2 tablespoons sugar
2 tablespoons cider vinegar
1 teaspoon salt
½ teaspoon fresh ground black pepper

1 package chicken flavored Ramen noodles, omitting spice packet
1 (10-ounce) package finely shredded cabbage (about 4 cups)
1 cup drained canned mandarin oranges
4 green onions, sliced into thin rounds
½ cup slivered almonds, toasted

In a small bowl, whisk together canola oil, sugar, vinegar, salt, and pepper. Whisk to combine well.

Break Ramen noodles into bite-size pieces and place in a medium serving bowl. Add cabbage, oranges, and onions. Toss with dressing. Garnish with almonds and serve.

Per serving: 129 calories; 11 grams carbohydrate; 2 grams fiber; 6 grams fat; 1 gram saturated fat; 2 grams protein; 267 milligrams sodium; 0 milligrams cholesterol; 30 milligrams calcium.

• •

Broccoli Slaw
Makes 4 servings.

Skip the overcooked broccoli spears for a more interesting take on this extremely nutritious vegetable.

¼ cup low-fat plain Greek yogurt
¼ cup reduced-fat mayonnaise
3 tablespoons cider vinegar
2 teaspoons sugar
Fresh ground black pepper, to taste
½ cup finely-diced red onion (about 1/2 a medium onion)
¼ cup dried cranberries
1 (16-ounce) bag shredded broccoli

In a large bowl, whisk together the yogurt, mayonnaise, vinegar, sugar, and pepper. Add the onion, cranberries, and broccoli; toss to coat. Chill until ready to serve.

Per serving: 124 calories; 22 grams carbohydrate; 4 grams fiber; 4 grams fat; 1 gram saturated fat; 4 grams protein; 150 milligrams sodium; 5 milligrams cholesterol; 90 milligrams calcium.

Mock Mashed Potatoes

Makes 4 servings.

Don't tell the cauliflower-haters what's in this creamy side dish. They wouldn't believe you, anyway!

2 cups chopped raw cauliflower
1 tablespoon trans-fat free tub margarine
¼ cup grated Parmesan cheese
½ cup low-fat (1%) milk
¼ cup chopped fresh parsley, or 2 tablespoons dried parsley

Steam or microwave cauliflower until very tender. Place cooked cauliflower, margarine, cheese, and milk in a food processor. Pulse until mixture reaches desired consistency, adding more milk, if necessary.

Transfer to a serving bowl. Stir in parsley.

Per serving: 73 calories; 4 grams carbohydrate; 1 gram fiber; 4 grams fat; 2 grams saturated fat; 4 grams protein; 147 milligrams sodium; 7 milligrams cholesterol; 120 milligrams calcium.

Crispy Chickpeas

Makes 4 servings.

Beans are the vegetable with the most protein and fiber, which makes them a perfect snack.

1 (15-ounce) can chickpeas (garbanzo beans), drained and rinsed
2 tablespoons olive oil
1 teaspoon ground cumin

Preheat oven to 400°F.

In a medium bowl, combine all ingredients, tossing to coat beans completely. Spread beans in a single layer on a rimmed baking sheet.

Bake for 20 minutes. Stir beans, and bake for another 20 minutes. Allow to cool before eating.

Per serving: 185 calories; 24 grams carbohydrate; 5 grams fiber; 8 grams fat; 1 gram saturated fat; 5 grams protein; 314 milligrams sodium; 0 milligrams cholesterol; 30 milligrams calcium.

• •

Roasted Baby Carrots and Red Onion with Rosemary
Makes 4 servings.

Roasting brings out the natural flavor of vegetables and reduces the amount of added fat and salt you need to make them taste great.

1 (1-pound) bag baby carrots
2 medium red onions, peeled, cut lengthwise into 12 wedges
2 tablespoons oil
1 tablespoon balsamic vinegar
1 tablespoon fresh chopped rosemary or 1 teaspoon dried rosemary
½ teaspoon salt
Fresh ground black pepper, if desired

Preheat oven to 400°F.

In a large bowl, toss together the carrots, onion, oil, vinegar, and rosemary. Spread in a single layer on large rimmed baking sheet. Sprinkle with salt and pepper. Bake for 20 minutes, or until vegetables are tender.

Per serving: 68 calories; 16 grams carbohydrate; 4 grams fiber; 0 grams fat; 0 grams saturated fat; 2 grams protein; 370 milligrams sodium; 0 milligrams cholesterol; 50 milligrams calcium.

• •

Shredded Beet Salad
Makes 4 servings.

Yes, you can eat beets raw. And boy, are they delicious.

5 medium raw beets, peeled
¼ cup sherry vinegar
2 teaspoons Dijon mustard
2 tablespoons olive oil
2 tablespoons fresh chopped chives

Using a grater, shred the beets. Place beets in a large serving bowl. In a small bowl, whisk vinegar, mustard, oil, and chives. Add to the beets, tossing to coat completely.

Per serving: 114 calories; 12 grams carbohydrate; 4 grams fiber; 7 grams fat; 1 gram saturated fat; 2 grams protein; 124 milligrams sodium; 0 milligrams cholesterol; 20 milligrams calcium.

Kale Chips
Makes 4 servings.

Here's a fun way to work in dark green leafy vegetables.

1 bunch kale (about 5 cups raw kale)
1 tablespoon olive oil
½ teaspoon salt

Preheat oven to 375°F.

Wash and dry kale. Remove tough stems. Tear kale into 2-inch pieces. Place kale in a large bowl. Add olive oil and toss to coat kale completely with the oil. Divide the kale between two baking sheets and spread it out into a single layer. Sprinkle with salt. Bake for 10 to 12 minutes or until the edges of the kale begins to brown.

Per serving: 72 calories; 8 grams carbohydrate; 2 grams fiber; 4 grams fat; 1 gram saturated fat; 3 grams protein; 327 milligrams sodium; 0 milligrams cholesterol; 110 milligrams calcium.

Spicy Sweet Potato Wedges
Makes 4 servings.

Cayenne pepper provides a kick in this spicy take on sweet potatoes.

4 medium raw sweet potatoes, peeled
1 tablespoon olive oil
1 tablespoon dark brown sugar
¼ teaspoon cayenne pepper
¼ teaspoon salt

Preheat oven to 400°F. Coat a large baking sheet with cooking spray.

Cut potatoes lengthwise into 1-inch wedges.

In a large bowl, combine oil, sugar, pepper, and salt. Add sweet potatoes and toss to coat completely.

Arrange sweet potatoes in a single layer on baking sheet. Roast for 15 minutes. Toss and bake for another 10 to 15 minutes or until golden brown.

Per serving: 154 calories; 29 grams carbohydrate; 4 grams fiber; 3 grams fat; 0 grams saturated fat; 2 grams protein; 218 milligrams sodium; 0 milligrams cholesterol; 401 milligrams calcium.

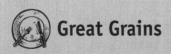 **Great Grains**

Nearly every one of us needs to eat more whole grains. Go beyond the traditional choices and try these easy-to-prepare recipes to work in more whole grains.

Farro Salad with Roasted Asparagus and Dried Cherries
Makes 5 servings.

Farro is a quick-cooking grain that's versatile and easy to use.

1 cup farro, uncooked
1½ cups low-sodium chicken or vegetable broth
1 bunch fresh asparagus
4 teaspoons olive oil
1 tablespoon balsamic vinegar
¼ teaspoon fresh ground black pepper
½ teaspoon dried thyme
¼ cup dried cherries
¼ cup feta cheese (1 ounce)

Preheat oven to 400°F.

Rinse farro. In a medium saucepan, combine farro and broth. Bring to a low boil for 15 to 20 minutes or until chewy.

Trim tough ends of asparagus. Cut asparagus into 1-inch pieces. Place asparagus in medium bowl. Add oil, vinegar, pepper, and thyme, and toss to coat asparagus completely. Place on baking sheet. Cook for 8 to 10 minutes or until just fork-tender.

In a medium serving bowl, combine cooked farro, cooked asparagus, dried cherries, and feta cheese. Toss to mix well.

Per serving (1 cup): 237 calories; 36 grams carbohydrate; 6 grams fiber; 7 grams fat; 2 grams saturated fat; 10 grams protein; 114 milligrams sodium; 7 milligrams cholesterol; 210 milligrams calcium.

Peanut Butter Noodles with Carrots and Broccoli
Makes 5 servings.

Turn this fun dish into an entrée by adding cubed tofu or cooked, shredded chicken.

8 ounces whole-wheat spaghetti, uncooked
3 tablespoons canola or vegetable oil
⅓ cup creamy peanut butter
3 tablespoons low-sodium soy sauce
2 tablespoons lime juice (about the amount in one lime)
1 tablespoon honey
2 tablespoons rice wine vinegar
1 cup raw grated carrots
2 cups cooked chopped broccoli florets
¼ to ½ teaspoon red pepper flakes (optional)
2 scallions, sliced into thin rounds

Cook spaghetti according to package directions. When done, rinse well with cold running water, and reserve.

While the pasta is cooking, combine the oil, peanut butter, soy sauce, lime juice, honey and vinegar in a large serving bowl. Using a whisk, mix until smooth. Add the spaghetti, carrots, broccoli, and red pepper flakes and toss to coat the noodle mixture completely. Garnish with scallions and serve.

Per serving (1 cup): 199 calories; 24 grams carbohydrate; 4 grams fiber; 11 grams fat; 1 gram saturated fat; 5 grams protein; 377 milligrams sodium; 0 milligrams cholesterol; 50 milligrams calcium.

Confetti Couscous
Makes 2½ cups.

Couscous, ready in minutes, provides an interesting alternative to rice.

¾ cup whole-wheat couscous, uncooked
1 cup water or low-sodium chicken or vegetable broth
½ teaspoon salt (omit if using broth)
2 teaspoons trans-fat free tub margarine
1 cup frozen diced carrots and peas, defrosted and warmed

In medium saucepan, bring water or broth, salt, and margarine to just a boil. Stir in couscous. Cover. Remove from heat. Let stand for five minutes. Fluff couscous lightly with a fork. Add carrots and peas; combine.

Per serving (½ cup cooked, using water and salt): 127 calories; 2 grams carbohydrate; 3 grams fiber; 2 grams fat; 0 grams saturated fat; 4 grams protein; 307 milligrams sodium; 0 milligrams cholesterol; 20 milligrams calcium.

• •

Pistachio Quinoa
Makes 3 servings.

Quinoa packs protein, which sets it apart from most other grains.

1 cup quinoa, uncooked
2 cups water
2 tablespoons olive oil
½ teaspoon salt
¼ cup chopped fresh parsley
¼ cup chopped unsalted pistachios
2 tablespoons lemon juice

In medium saucepan, combine quinoa, water, olive oil, and salt. Bring quinoa mixture to a boil, then reduce heat, cover, and simmer for about 15 minutes or until quinoa is still chewy.

Remove from heat. Add parsley, pistachios, and lemon juice to quinoa and toss to mix completely.

Per serving (1 cup): 173 calories; 20 grams carbohydrate; 3 grams fiber; 9 grams fat; 1 gram saturated fat; 5 grams protein; 196 milligrams sodium; 0 milligrams cholesterol; 20 milligrams calcium.

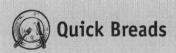 **Quick Breads**

Make healthy muffins and bread ahead of time and freeze for later in the week when time gets tight.

Pumpkin Raisin Pancakes
Makes 6 servings (3 pancakes per serving).

Pumpkin and raisins are brimming with good nutrition in this twist on classic pancakes. Each serving provides two-thirds of the calcium in a glass of milk.

2 cups plain low-fat yogurt
¼ cup plus 1 tablespoon sugar
1²/₃ cups all-purpose flour
1 teaspoon baking soda
1 teaspoon cinnamon
½ teaspoon ground nutmeg
1 cup low-fat (1%) milk
2 tablespoons trans fat–free tub margarine, melted
1 large egg
½ cup canned pumpkin
½ cup California raisins

In a small bowl, mix the yogurt with ¼ cup of the sugar. Set aside. In a large bowl, combine 1 tablespoon of sugar with the flour, baking soda, cinnamon, and nutmeg.

In a medium bowl, combine the milk, margarine, egg, pumpkin, raisins, and yogurt-sugar mixture, stirring well. Add the wet ingredients to the dry ingredients in the large bowl. Stir until batter is moist and free of lumps.

Lightly coat a griddle or a skillet with nonstick cooking spray and heat to low to medium heat. Using a ¼ cup measure, pour the batter onto the hot griddle. Cook until the bubbles begin to burst, then flip and cook until golden brown.

Per serving: 302 calories; 57 grams carbohydrate; 2 grams fiber; 4 grams fat; 2 grams saturated fat; 11 grams protein; 305 milligrams sodium; 42 milligrams cholesterol; 220 milligrams calcium.

Sweet Potato, Pecan, and Cranberry Muffins
Makes 12 muffins.

These muffins are a great way to use leftover cooked sweet potato.

1 cup all-purpose flour
½ cup sugar
¾ teaspoon baking powder
1 teaspoon cinnamon
½ teaspoon salt
½ cup dried cranberries
½ cup chopped pecans
½ cup mashed cooked sweet potato
½ cup low-fat buttermilk
¼ cup canola or vegetable oil
1 large egg

Preheat oven to 375°F.

In a large bowl, combine flour, sugar, baking powder, cinnamon, and salt. Stir in cranberries and pecans.

In a medium bowl, combine sweet potato, buttermilk, oil, and egg; mix well. Add sweet potato mixture to dry ingredients, and stir until dry ingredients are just moistened.

Line 12 muffin pans with paper muffin cups, and divide batter equally among muffin cups. Fill muffin cups half full. Bake for 12 to 15 minutes or until a toothpick inserted in the center comes out clean. Remove muffins from pans and cool on a wire rack.

Per serving (1 muffin): 174 calories; 23 grams carbohydrate; 1 gram fiber; 8 grams fat; 1 gram saturated fat; 3 grams protein; 147 milligrams sodium; 18 milligrams cholesterol; 40 milligrams calcium.

Applesauce Walnut Bread

Makes 2 loaves (24 servings).

Whole-wheat flour and oatmeal lend whole grain goodness, and the walnuts contribute heart-healthy fat and other beneficial nutrients. Unsweetened applesauce means less added fat and sugar.

2 cups all-purpose flour
1 cup whole-wheat flour
1 tablespoon baking powder
1 tablespoon ground cinnamon
1 teaspoon salt
1 teaspoon baking soda
2 cups one-minute oatmeal, uncooked
1 cup light brown sugar, packed
1½ cups golden California raisins
1½ cups chopped walnuts
2½ cups unsweetened applesauce
⅔ cup canola or vegetable oil
4 large eggs
½ cup low-fat (1%) milk

Preheat the oven to 350°F. Lightly grease and flour two loaf pans.

In a large bowl, combine the flours, baking powder, cinnamon, salt, baking soda, oatmeal, brown sugar, raisins, and walnuts. Stir until well combined.

In a medium bowl, whisk together the applesauce, canola oil, eggs, and milk.

Add the applesauce mixture to the flour mixture and stir until the dry ingredients are moistened.

Fill the prepared pans with the batter, dividing evenly. Bake for 30 to 35 minutes or until a toothpick inserted in the center comes out clean. Let bread cool before slicing.

Per serving (¹/₁₂ loaf): 218 calories; 38 grams carbohydrate; 3 grams fiber; 6 grams fat; 1 gram saturated fat; 5 grams protein; 244 milligrams sodium; 36 milligrams cholesterol; 90 milligrams calcium.

Better For You Blueberry Muffins
Makes 18 muffins.

1½ cups whole-wheat flour
½ cups plus 1 tablespoon all-purpose flour
½ cup sugar
4 teaspoons baking powder
¼ teaspoon baking soda
1 teaspoon salt
1 teaspoon ground cinnamon
1 large egg
¼ cup canola oil
1 teaspoon vanilla extract
1 cup fat-free plain Greek yogurt
½ cup low-fat (1%) milk
1 cup fresh or frozen blueberries (not defrosted)

Preheat oven to 375°F.

In a large bowl, whisk together whole-wheat flour, ½ cup all-purpose flour, sugar, baking powder, baking soda, salt, and cinnamon.

In a medium bowl, whisk together egg, oil, vanilla, yogurt, and milk.

In a small bowl, toss the blueberries with 1 tablespoon flour until lightly coated. Add to egg mixture, then add the egg mixture to the flour mixture.

Using a spatula, fold ingredients together just until dry ingredients are moistened. Line 18 muffin pans with paper muffin cups, and divide batter equally among muffin cups.

Bake for 8 to 12 minutes or until a toothpick inserted in the center comes out clean.

Per serving (1 muffin): 105 calories; 16 grams carbohydrate; 1 gram fiber; 4 grams fat; 0 grams saturated fat; 3 grams protein; 270 milligrams sodium; 12 milligrams cholesterol; 100 milligrams calcium.

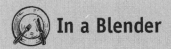

In a Blender

Each of these scrumptious concoctions is a great way to drink good nutrition, but don't take these recipes as gospel. Personalize your drink by substituting a fortified soy beverage or soy yogurt, and using whatever fruit you have on hand. Nearly all of the recipes combine a serving of fruit and dairy.

Cherry Vanilla Freeze
Makes 1 serving.

Use frozen peaches if you don't have cherries.

¾ cup frozen sweet cherries, pitted
1 cup plain low-fat yogurt
2 ice cubes
½ teaspoon vanilla extract

Combine all ingredients in a blender or food processor. Blend. Pour into a tall glass and drink immediately.

Per serving: 227 calories; 36 grams carbohydrate; 2 grams fiber; 4 grams fat; 2 grams saturated fat; 14 grams protein; 171 milligrams sodium; 15 milligrams cholesterol; 460 milligrams calcium.

• •

Almond Delight
Makes 1 serving.

Any nut or seed butter will do, but almond butter is yummy!

1 banana, peeled
1 cup plain nonfat Greek yogurt
2 tablespoons almond butter
3 ice cubes

Combine all ingredients in a blender or food processor. Blend. Pour into a tall glass and drink immediately.

Per serving: 344 calories; 49 grams carbohydrate; 4 grams fiber; 10 grams fat; 1 gram saturated fat; 18 grams protein; 262 milligrams sodium; 5 milligrams cholesterol; 540 milligrams calcium.

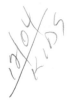

Cinnamon Pumpkin Smoothie

Makes 1 serving.

Cinnamon brings out the natural sweetness of pumpkin, so you don't need much added sugar.

½ cup fat-free milk
½ cup canned pumpkin
2 teaspoons brown sugar
½ teaspoon vanilla extract
pinch ground cinnamon
2 ice cubes

Combine all ingredients in a blender or food processor. Blend. Pour into a tall glass and drink immediately.

Per serving: 106 calories; 22 grams carbohydrate; 4 grams fiber; 0 grams fat; 0 grams saturated fat; 5 grams protein; 59 milligrams sodium; 2 milligrams cholesterol; 190 milligrams calcium.

Chocolate Banana Sipper

Makes 1 serving.

Chocolate and bananas are especially appealing, and good for you, too.

1 medium banana, peeled
8 ounces low-fat (1%) milk
1 tablespoon unsweetened cocoa powder
1 teaspoon sugar
2 ice cubes

Combine all ingredients in a blender or food processor. Blend. Pour into a tall glass and drink immediately.

Per serving: 223 calories; 44 grams carbohydrate; 3 grams fiber; 3 grams fat; 2 grams saturated fat; 10 grams protein; 109 milligrams sodium; 12 milligrams cholesterol; 300 milligrams calcium.

Orange Mango Cooler
Makes 1 serving.

Mango is brimming with vitamin C and beta carotene (the building block of vitamin A in the body) and provides more than 20 different vitamins and minerals. What's not to love?

½ cup frozen mango chunks
¾ cup plain fat-free yogurt
½ teaspoon vanilla extract
¼ cup orange juice

Combine all ingredients in a blender or food processor. Blend. Pour into a tall glass and drink immediately.

Per serving: 212 calories; 41 grams carbohydrate; 2 grams fiber; 1 gram fat; 0 grams saturated fat; 12 grams protein; 144 milligrams sodium; 4 milligrams cholesterol; 390 milligrams calcium.

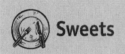 **Sweets**

MyPlate and the 2010 Dietary Guidelines recommend limiting added solid fats and sugars, but they don't advise you to completely avoid them. Everyone has room for sweets, if they so desire. These recipes were designed to pack in good nutrition while keeping calories, fat, and sugar to a minimum.

Red Velvet Brownies
Makes 12 servings.

Try your best not to divulge the secret of these moist, and colorful, chocolate treats.

4 ounces semi-sweet chocolate (squares or chips)
2 tablespoons unsweetened cocoa powder
¾ cup all-purpose flour
2 teaspoons baking powder
¼ teaspoon salt
½ cup trans-fat free tub margarine

⅓ cup sugar

2 large eggs

1½ teaspoons vanilla extract

¾ cup pureed cooked beets *(Note: One 15-ounce can of no-salt-added cooked beets makes 1 cup beet puree.)*

Preheat oven to 350°F. Grease an 8- x 8-inch baking pan. In a medium microwavable bowl, melt chocolate. Add cocoa powder and mix well.

In a medium bowl, combine flour, baking powder, and salt.

In a large mixing bowl, cream margarine with sugar. Add eggs, one at a time, until the mixture is creamy. Add vanilla, melted chocolate mixture, beets, and flour mixture. Mix until dry ingredients are combined, but do not overmix.

Pour batter into prepared pan. Bake for 20 to 25 minutes, or until a knife inserted in the center comes out clean.

Per serving: 187 calories; 21 grams carbohydrate; 1 gram fiber; 11 grams fat; 3 grams saturated fat; 3 grams protein; 272 milligrams sodium; 37 milligrams cholesterol; 70 milligrams calcium.

• •

Roasted Pineapple

Makes 4 servings.

Roasted pineapple is an elegant treat that's easy to prepare and sure to impress.

2 tablespoons dark brown sugar

1 teaspoon ground cinnamon

1 whole pineapple (about 2½ to 3 pounds)

Heat broiler. In a small bowl, combine sugar and cinnamon.

Trim leaves and bud end from pineapple. Using a sharp serated knife, cut pineapple into ½-inch slices. Place slices in a single layer on a baking sheet. Sprinkle with sugar mixture.

Broil for 10 to 15 minutes. Turn slices over and broil for 5 to 10 minutes more, or until pineapple is tender and golden brown.

Per serving: 110 calories; 29 grams carbohydrate; 2 grams fiber; 0 grams fat; 0 grams saturated fat; 1 gram protein; 4 milligrams sodium; 0 milligrams cholesterol; 30 milligrams calcium.

S'Mores Trail Mix

Makes 1 serving.

This is a fun treat for kids, made healthier with raisins.

2 graham cracker squares, broken into pieces
¼ cup mini marshmallows
2 tablespoons California raisins
2 tablespoons chocolate chips

In a small bowl, combine all ingredients. Store in an airtight container if not eating immediately.

Per serving: 198 calories; 36 grams carbohydrate; 1 gram fiber; 6 grams fat; 3 grams saturated fat; 3 grams protein; 103 milligrams sodium; 3 milligrams cholesterol; 40 milligrams calcium.

Honey Blueberry Sauce

Makes 2 cups.

A delicious addition to plain fat-free yogurt, fat-free frozen yogurt, or cooked oatmeal.

4 cups fresh or frozen blueberries
½ cup honey
¼ cup lemon juice

Stir blueberries, honey, and lemon juice together in a medium saucepan. Bring to a boil; reduce heat to maintain a simmer and cook, stirring occasionally, until thickened, about 15 minutes. Let cool for 10 minutes; serve warm, if desired. (Tastes great cold on whole-grain toast topped with low-fat cottage cheese.)

Per serving (2 tablespoons): 86 calories; 23 grams carbohydrate; 1 gram fiber; 0 grams fat; 0 grams saturated fat; 0 grams protein; 1 milligram sodium; 0 milligrams cholesterol; 0 milligrams calcium.

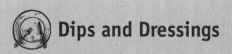

Dips and Dressings

Dips and dressings that you buy at the store can be loaded with sodium. These lower-salt options pack flavor, take just minutes to make, and keep for days.

Ranch Dressing
Makes 2 cups.

Buttermilk provides a slight tang in this perennial favorite.

½ cup buttermilk
¼ cup low-fat sour cream or plain low-fat Greek yogurt
2 tablespoons low-fat mayonnaise
2 tablespoons chopped fresh parsley, chives, or basil, or a combination
¼ teaspoon salt
¼ teaspoon fresh ground black pepper

In a small bowl, combine all ingredients. Mix well. Refrigerate.

Per serving (1 tablespoon): 8 calories; 1 gram carbohydrate; 0 grams fiber; 0 grams fat; 0 grams saturated fat; 0 grams protein; 52 milligrams sodium; 1 milligram cholesterol; 10 milligrams calcium.

• •

Zesty Vinaigrette
Makes 1 cup.

Honey balances the mustard and complex balsamic vinegar allows for less oil, and lowers fat levels.

¼ cup olive oil
½ cup balsamic vinegar
1 teaspoon Dijon mustard
2 teaspoons honey
1 teaspoon dried oregano

In a small bowl, combine all ingredients. Mix well. Refrigerate.

Per serving (1 tablespoon): 33 calories; 1 gram carbohydrate; 0 grams fiber; 3 grams fat; 0 grams saturated fat; 0 grams protein; 2 milligrams sodium; 0 milligrams cholesterol; 0 milligrams calcium.

Orange Ginger Dressing
Makes 1 cup.

OJ is not just for breakfast. It provides a fruit base in this Asian-inspired salad dressing.

½ cup orange juice
¼ cup canola oil
1 clove garlic, peeled and minced
2 green onions, thinly sliced
½ teaspoon fresh grated ginger

In a small bowl, combine all ingredients. Mix well. Refrigerate.

Per serving (1 tablespoon): 36 calories; 1 gram carbohydrate; 0 grams fiber; 4 grams fat; 0 grams saturated fat; 0 grams protein; 0 milligrams sodium; 0 milligrams cholesterol; 0 milligrams calcium.

Salsamole
Makes 2 cups.

Simple, nutritious, and delicious. Use as a dip or sandwich spread.

1 cup fresh tomato salsa
1 cup fresh guacamole
2 tablespoons lime juice
2 tablespoons chopped cilantro

Combine all ingredients in medium serving bowl. Refrigerate.

Per serving (¼ cup): 94 calories; 6 grams carbohydrate; 3 grams fiber; 8 grams; 1 gram saturated fat; 2 grams protein; 229 milligrams sodium; 0 milligrams cholesterol; 20 milligrams calcium.

Mango and Black Bean Salsa
Makes 2½ cups.

High in fiber, and pretty to look at, this salsa tastes even better the next day.

2 cups diced fresh mango
2 cups black beans, rinsed and drained, if canned
½ cup diced red onion
1 to 2 tablespoons finely chopped, seeded jalapeno pepper
2 tablespoons chopped fresh cilantro
2 tablespoons lime juice
½ teaspoon salt

In a medium bowl, combine all ingredients. Refrigerate.

Per serving (¼ cup): 69 calories; 14 grams carbohydrate; 4 grams fiber; 0 grams fat; 0 grams saturated fat; 3 grams protein; 199 milligrams sodium; 0 milligrams cholesterol; 10 milligrams calcium.

Creamy Cucumber Dressing
Makes 2 cups.

Add a pinch of garlic powder for even more flavor.

1 cup plain low-fat Greek yogurt or low-fat sour cream
½ cup cucumber, peeled and seeded, finely chopped
3 tablespoons rice wine vinegar
⅛ teaspoon fresh ground pepper
¼ teaspoon salt

In a small bowl, combine all ingredients. Mix well. Refrigerate.

Per serving (1 tablespoon): 11 calories; 0 grams carbohydrate; 0 grams fiber; 1 gram fat; 1 gram saturated fat; 0 grams protein; 40 milligrams sodium; 3 milligrams cholesterol; 10 milligrams calcium.

Introduction

U.S. Department of Agriculture and U.S. Department of Health and Human Services. Dietary Guidelines for Americans 2010. 7th Edition. Washington, D.C.: U.S. Government Printing Office, December 2010. www.cnpp.usda.gov/dietaryguidelines.htm

U.S. Department of Agriculture. MyPlate. www.ChooseMyPlate.gov

Chapter One

Mozaffarian, D., et al. Changes in Diet and Lifestyle and Long-Term Weight Gain in Women and Men. *New England Journal of Medicine* 364 (25):2392-2404, 2011. www.nejm.org/doi/full/10.1056/NEJMoa1014296

Vander Wal, J.S., et al. Egg Breakfast Enhances Weight Loss. *International Journal of Obesity* 32(10):1545-1551, 2008. www.nature.com/ijo/journal/vaop/ncurrent/abs/ijo2008130a.html

Wing, R.R., and Phelan, S. Long-Term Weight Loss Maintenance. *American Journal of Clinical Nutrition* 82(suppl):222S-225S, 2005. www.ajcn.org/content/82/1/222S.abstract

Racette, S.B., et al. Influence of Weekend Lifestyle Patterns on Body Weight. *Obesity* 16(8):1826-1830, 2008. www.nature.com/oby/journal/v16/n8/abs/oby2008320a.html

Chapter Two

U. S. Department of Health and Human Services. 2008 Physical Activity Guidelines for Americans. http://www.health.gov/PAGuidelines/

Mozaffarian, D., et al. Changes in Diet and Lifestyle and Long-Term Weight Gain in Women and Men. *New England Journal of Medicine* 364 (25):2392-2404, 2011. www.nejm.org/doi/full/10.1056/NEJMoa1014296

American Academy of Pediatrics, Committee on Public Education. Children, Adolescents, and Television. *Pediatrics* 107(2): 423-426, 2001.

American Dietetic Association and American Dietetic Association Foundation. The State of Family Nutrition and Physical Activity: Are We Making Progress? www.eatright.org/foundation/fnpa/ADA

Piernas, C., and Popkin, B.M. Trends In Snacking Among U.S. Children. *Health Affairs* 29:398-404, 2011. content.healthaffairs.org/content/29/3/398. abstract?related-urls=yes&legid=healthaff;29/3/398

Rasmussen, K.M. and Yaktine, A.L. Editors; Committee to Reexamine IOM Pregnancy Weight Guidelines; Institute of Medicine; National Research Council. Weight Gain During Pregnancy: Reexamining the Guidelines. Washington, D.C.: National Academy Press, 2009.

Chapter Three

U. S. Department of Health and Human Services. 2008 Physical Activity Guidelines for Americans. http://www.health.gov/PAGuidelines/

Chapter Four

U.S. Department of Agriculture and U.S. Department of Health and Human Services. Dietary Guidelines for Americans 2010. 7th Edition. Washington, D.C.: U.S. Government Printing Office, December 2010. www.cnpp.usda.gov/dietaryguidelines.htm

Institute of Medicine, Food and Nutrition Board. Dietary Reference Intakes for Calcium and Vitamin D. Washington, D.C.: National Academy Press, 2010.

Institute of Medicine. Dietary Reference Intakes for Water, Potassium, Sodium, Chloride, and Sulfate. Washington, D.C.: National Academy Press, 2004.

Institute of Medicine. Dietary Reference Intakes for Energy, Carbohydrate, Fiber, Fat, Fatty Acids, Cholesterol, Protein, and Amino Acids. Washington, D.C.: National Academy Press, 2002.

Chapter Six

Institute of Medicine. Dietary Reference Intakes for Water, Potassium, Sodium, Chloride, and Sulfate. Washington, D.C.: National Academy Press, 2004.

American Heart Association. Know Your Fats. www.heart.org/HEARTORG/Conditions/Cholesterol/PreventionTreatmentofHighCholesterol/Know-Your-Fats_UCM_305628_Article.jsp

Chapter Seven

U.S. Food and Drug Administration. What Fish Should Pregnant Women Avoid? www.fda.gov/Food/FoodSafety/Product-SpecificInformation/Seafood/ConsumerInformationAboutSeafood/ucm122607.htm

U.S. Food and Drug Administration. Summary of Qualified Health Claims Subject to Enforcement Discretion, Qualified Claims About Cardiovascular Disease Risk, Nuts & Heart Disease. www.fda.gov/Food/LabelingNutrition/LabelClaims/QualifiedHealthClaims/ucm073992.htm#nuts

Institute of Medicine. Dietary Reference Intakes for Energy, Carbohydrate, Fiber, Fat, Fatty Acids, Cholesterol, Protein, and Amino Acids. Washington, D.C.: National Academy Press, 2002.

Chapter Eight

Johnson, R.K., et al. Dietary Sugars Intake and Cardiovascular Health, A Scientific Statement From the American Heart Association. *Circulation* 120:1011-1020, 2009. circ.ahajournals.org/content/120/11/1011.full.pdf

Institute of Medicine. Dietary Reference Intakes for Water, Potassium, Sodium, Chloride, and Sulfate. Washington, D.C.: National Academy Press, 2004.

Health Canada. Caffeine. http://www.hc-sc.gc.ca/hl-vs/iyh-vsv/food-aliment/caffeine-eng.php

Resources

American Dietetic Association
www.eatright.org

Dietitians of Canada
www.dietitians.ca

Dietary Guidelines for Americans, 2010
www.cnpp.usda.gov/dietaryguidelines.htm

MyPlate
www.ChooseMyPlate.gov

Nutrition Blog Network: A collection of blogs written by registered dietitians.
nutritionblognetwork.com

U.S. Food and Drug Administration, Center for Food Safety and Nutrition,
www.cfsan.fda.gov; Food Information Line, 1-888-SAFEFOOD

Recommended Reading

Read It Before You Eat It, How to Decode Food Labels and Make the Healthiest Choice Every Time, by Bonnie Taub-Dix, MA, RD, CDN. Plume, 2010.

7-Day Menu Planner for Dummies, by Susan Nicholson, RD/LD. Wiley Publishing, 2010.

The Calorie Counter for Dummies, by Rosanne Rust, MS, RD, LDN and Meri Raffetto, RD, LDN. Wiley Publishing, 2010.

Restaurant Calorie Counter for Dummies, by Rosanne Rust, MS, RD, LDN and Meri Raffetto, RD, LDN. Wiley Publishing, 2011.

No Whine with Dinner, 150 Healthy, Kid-Tested Recipes from The Meal Makeover Moms, by Liz Weiss, MS, RD and Janice Newell Bissex, MS, RD. M3Press, 2011.

Nutrition at Your Fingertips, by Elisa Zied, MS, RD, CDN. Alpha, 2009.

Eat Right When Time Is Tight, 150 Slim-Down Strategies and No-Cook Food Fixes, by Patricia Bannan, MS, RD. NorLightsPress, 2010.

Go UnDiet, by Gloria Tsang, RD. Health Castle Media, 2011.

Mindless Eating, Why We Eat More Than We Think, by Brian Wansink, PhD. Bantam Books, 2006.

101 Optimal Life Foods, by Dave Grotto, RD, LDN. Bantam Books, 2010

Guide to Healthy Restaurants: What to eat in America's most popular chain restaurants, by Hope Warshaw, MMSc, RD, CDE. American Diabetes Association, 2009.

The Flexitarian Diet: The Mostly Vegetarian Way to Lose Weight, Be Healthier, Prevent Disease, and Add Years to Your Life, by Dawn Jackson Blatner, RD, LDN. McGraw-Hill, 2010.

fruits and vegetables, 59-62
  how to eat more, 61-62
  recommended servings of, 59-60

G

gender and calorie needs, 6
grains, refined, 70-71

H

Haddock In a Packet, 128
heavy drinking of alcohol, 106
hydrogenated fat, 79

I

iodine, 73-74
iodized salt, 73-74
iron, 29-30
  heme, 30
  non-heme, 30
iron-rich foods, 30

J

juice, nutrition of, 103

K

Kale Chips, 143
kitchen staples shopping list, 116

L

Lasagna, Almost, 122
low-calorie sweeteners, 70

M

Mashed Potatoes, Mock 141
meal planning, 115-116
mercury, 94
Metabolic syndrome, 35
milk, 111
  benefits of lower-fat, 111
  recommended servings of, 58
milk fat, 68
Minestrone in Minutes, 138
mixed alcoholic drinks and calories, 105
monk fruit, 70
monosaturated fat, 80-81

Muffins, Sweet Potato, Pecan,
  and Cranberry, 148
Muffins, Better for You Blueberry, 150
muscle-strengthening activity, 38

N

Noodles with Carrots and Broccoli,
  Peanut Butter, 145
nutrient-rich foods, 56-64
Nutrition Facts label, 10, 80
nuts, 90

O

oils, 81-83, 91
  amounts of in fatty foods, 83
omega-3s, 80-81
  recommended servings of, 95
  supplements, 81
overeating triggers, 11-16
overweight children, 19-21

P

Pancakes, Pumpkin Raisin, 147
Panini, Chicken, Apple, and Cheese, 133
Pasta Recipes
  Almost Lasagna, 122
  Confetti Couscous, 145
  *Pasta with Sundried Tomatoes, Spinach,
    and Garbanzo Beans,* 127
  *Peanut Butter Noodles with Carrots and
    Broccoli,* 145
  Ramen Noodle Salad, 139
  Roasted Shrimp and Orzo Salad, 125
Pasta with Sundried Tomatoes, Spinach,
  and Garbanzo Beans, 127
physical activity, 5
  a plan for, 40
  amount needed, 35-39
  amount needed for children, 41-42
  benefits of, 34-35
  for children, 23-24, 40-42
  for the family, 42
  *solutions to getting adequate
    amounts of,* 43-44
  type of, 35-39
Pineapple, Roasted, 154

Cinnamon Pumpkin Smoothie, 152
Orange Mango Cooler, 153
snacks, for children, 25-27
sodium, 72-75
   high blood pressure and, 74
   recommendations, 72
   reducing, 74-75
sodium-rich foods, 73
SoFAS daily calorie limits, 102
solid fat, 79, 91
   added sugars and, 67-70
   examples of, 69
Soup and Stew Recipes
   Chocolate Chili, 121
   Cream of Squash Soup, 139
   Minestrone in Minutes, 138
   Slow Cooker Middle Eastern Stew, 118
sources of added sugars, 101
spices, 75-76
sports drinks, 108
Squash Soup, Cream of, 139
Steak Tacos with Salsamole, 120
Stew, Slow Cooker Middle Eastern, 118
Stir-Fry, Pork, Asparagus, and Cashew, 123
sugar levels in beverages, 102
sugary beverages, 101
Sweet Potato Wedges, Spicy, 143

T
Tilapia Tacos, 124
tomatoes, 60
Trail Mix, S'mores, 155
trans fats, 79-80
triglycerides, 80
Tuna Patties on Whole-Wheat English
   Muffins, 135
Turkey Burgers, 136

U
unsaturated fat, 80-81

V
vegan diets, nutrients lacking in, 98
Vegetable Side Dish Recipes
   Broccoli Slaw, 140

Crispy Chickpeas, 141
Kale Chips, 143
Mock Mashed Potatoes, 141
Minestrone in Minutes, 138
Portabello Mushroom Parmesan, 137
Ramen Noodle Salad, 139
*Roasted Baby Carrots and Red Onion
   with Rosemary,* 142
Shredded Beet Salad, 142
*Smashed Yukon Gold Potatoes with
   Garlic and Chives,* 137
Spicy Sweet Potato Wedges, 143
vegetarian and vegan eating plans and
   protein, 98
Vegetarian Main Dish Recipes
   Bean 'N Cheese Enchiladas, 127
   Egg and Artichoke Pie, 126
   Egg and Mushroom Pita Pocket, 131
   Eggs Florentine Wrap, 134
   *Pasta with Sundried Tomatoes, Spinach,
   and Garbanzo Beans,* 127
vitamin B12, 55-56
   requirements, 55
vitamin B12-rich foods, 56
vitamin D, 51-52
   requirements, 52
vitamin D-rich foods, 52

W
Walnut Bread, Applesauce, 149
water, 107-109
   benefits of, 107-108
   daily requirements of, 108
   in food, 108
weight loss, 3, 8-9
Whole-Grain Recipes
   Confetti Couscous, 145
   *Farro Salad with Roasted Asparagus
   and Dried Cherries,* 144
   *Peanut Butter Noodles with Carrots
   and Broccoli,* 145
   Pistachio Quinoa, 146
whole grains, 63-64
Wrap, Eggs Florentine, 134

Made in the USA
Charleston, SC
03 September 2011